TIPS AND TRICKS IN
TRAUMA MANAGEMENT

System requirement:
- **Windows XP or above**
- **Power DVD player (Software)**
- **Windows media player 11.0 version or above (Software)**

Accompanying DVD ROM is playable only in Computer and not in DVD player.

Kindly wait for few seconds for DVD to autorun. If it does not autorun then please do the following:
- Click on my computer
- Click the **CD/DVD drive** and after opening the drive, kindly double click the file **Jaypee**

DVD Contents

- **Surgery for lateral condyle humerus**
- **Surgery for lateral condyle-2**
- **Bracing of knee**
- **Below elbow plastering**

TIPS AND TRICKS IN
TRAUMA MANAGEMENT

Sejal G Shah MBBS MS(Orthopedic)
Senior Consulting Trauma and
Joint Replacement Surgeon
NISARG Orthopedic and Maternity Hospital
Vadodara, Gujarat, India

Formerly
Ex Assistant Professor
Department of Orthopedics
SBKS Medical College
Pipariya, Vadodara, Gujarat, India

JAYPEE BROTHERS MEDICAL PUBLISHERS (P) LTD

New Delhi • St Louis • Panama City • London

Published by
Jaypee Brothers Medical Publishers (P) Ltd

Corporate Office
4838/24, Ansari Road, Daryaganj, **New Delhi** 110 002, India
Phone: +91-11-43574357, Fax: +91-11-43574314

Offices in India

- **Ahmedabad**, e-mail: ahmedabad@jaypeebrothers.com
- **Bengaluru**, e-mail: bangalore@jaypeebrothers.com
- **Chennai**, e-mail: chennai@jaypeebrothers.com
- **Delhi**, e-mail: jaypee@jaypeebrothers.com
- **Hyderabad**, e-mail: hyderabad@jaypeebrothers.com
- **Kochi**, e-mail: kochi@jaypeebrothers.com
- **Kolkata**, e-mail: kolkata@jaypeebrothers.com
- **Lucknow**, e-mail: lucknow@jaypeebrothers.com
- **Mumbai**, e-mail: mumbai@jaypeebrothers.com
- **Nagpur**, e-mail: nagpur@jaypeebrothers.com

Overseas Offices

- **North America Office, USA**, Ph: 001-636-6279734
  e-mail: jaypee@jaypeebrothers.com, anjulav@jaypeebrothers.com
- **Central America Office, Panama City, Panama**, Ph: 001-507-317-0160
  e-mail: cservice@jphmedical.com, Website: www.jphmedical.com
- **Europe Office, UK**, Ph: +44 (0) 2031708910
  e-mail: info@jpmedpub.com

Tips and Tricks in Trauma Management

© 2011, Jaypee Brothers Medical Publishers

This book has been published in good faith that the material provided by author is original. Every effort is made to ensure accuracy of material, but the publisher, printer and author will not be held responsible for any inadvertent error(s). In case of any dispute, all legal matters are to be settled under Delhi jurisdiction only.

First Edition: 2011

ISBN 978-93-5025-032-7

Typeset at JPBMP typesetting unit

Printed at Rajkamal Electric Press, Kundli, Haryana.

To

My beloved grandfather (late) Dr Somalal K Shah
who taught me that
if we pursue what we want, we will get that one day.

My parents, my wife and my darling children
Who are my efficiency to bring proficiency into action.

Foreword

This treatise will provide valuable supplementation in the management of orthopedic trauma, which is contained in major fracture texts. There is growing need for this type of detailed "how to do it" guidance.

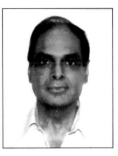

Successive global burden of disease and injury analysis documents the growing prevalence of road traffic injuries. Systems are evolving to the level where surgeons will be able to employ modern methods of management to avoid disabilities.

Trauma cuts short many productive lives. According to the American data, injury kills one person every six minutes and disabling injury occurs every two seconds. This is accentuated in rural setting where mortalities are 50% higher. The economic impact of trauma is significant and involves both direct costs of care and lost productivity.

More number of casualties are saved because of improvement in the understanding and management of a critically injured patient. Thus more number of orthopedic traumas has to be managed than before. It should be managed right from the site of injury to returning to his original workplace with little or no disability. The integrated trauma service concept enhances education and research as well as patient care.

Separating orthopedic trauma care from general or elective orthopedic practice has advantages for both. There are strong reasons and sound case to project orthopedic trauma management as a distinct specialty because specialization means a higher level of care. It is so much easier to teach and learn good habits early in surgical career than trying to unlearn bad habits later. This is precisely what author of this treatise must be having in mind.

VM Shah MS (Orthopedic)
VM Shah Hospital
Jamnagar, Gujarat, India

Preface

This is a small gesture and workmanship to craft a management of trauma in this jet life.

As it was difficult to understand, how, when and what to write, because this was first time in my life that I was handling a job of writing a book. Actually, idea of writing this book came through series of events which occurred in my life in the last 15 years, from my college days to flourishing practice that compelled me to write.

This book has unique feature as *Basics of Trauma Narrated in Stages of Trauma*, so that students to specialized doctors can understand, remember and apply it easily and appropriately in their practical traumatic life.

It is an immense pleasure to introduce my personal views and my practical experience what my eyes and brain learnt from my teachers, colleagues and others to share with you in form of a small handbook.

It has got beautiful live photographs, diagrammatic pictures, to the point 'steps to tips', and 'tracks to tricks' to offer each one of you for your own and better world today and tomorrow. Unnecessary theory material is excluded to make it more precise and ready for practical use.

Specialized section of specific trauma is designed to deal with particular person.

Rehabilitation, least attended part in our practice, is given utmost importance to get better functional outcome.

In fact, the word Doctor is derived from the Latin word 'Docere' means 'to teach'. It is very important that every doctor must be expert, trained, vigilant and accurate enough to be prepared in this unknown, undiagnosed, unwanted trauma to deal with.

I hope you would like this humble endeavor.

I wish you all a hassle free, successful and atraumatic life in this puzzling world.

Sejal G Shah

Acknowledgments

I have taken great efforts to write this book. However, it would not have been possible without kind support of many great people who have helped and supported me during writing and publishing of this book.

On this memorable moment of writing this book, I also would like to thank all who directly or indirectly involved with this book.

My deepest thanks to my wife Dr Shweta Shah, my sons Yug and Arnav, who helped me emotionally and morally encouraged me to pen my thoughts and experiences. She has taken pain to go through the book and make necessary corrections as and when needed.

I express my thanks to my doctors, teachers, colleagues, students, plastic surgeons, physiotherapists, my hospital staff who helped me to make a complete handbook.

I would like to express my deep sense of gratitude to Mr Tarun Duneja (Director-Publishing), Mr KK Raman (Production Manager), Mr Ashutosh Srivastava (Asstt. Editor) and the entire team of M/s Jaypee Brothers Medical Publishers (P) Ltd., New Delhi.

My special thanks to Dr VM Shah, renowned trauma surgeon for writing Foreword for this book.

And at last, I would like to thank almighty, God, and my patients for their kindness and their grace has made me what I am today.

Contents

Plate 1

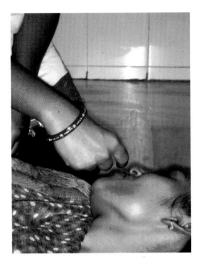

Fig. 3.6: Look, listen and feel for breathing

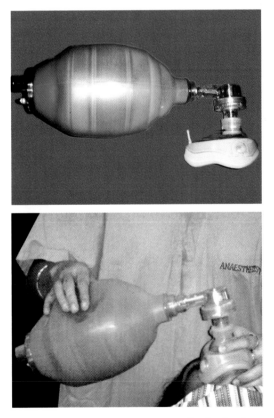

Fig. 3.7: Artificial ventilation (Ambu Bag)

Plate 2

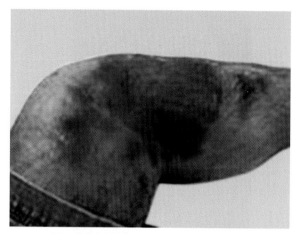

Fig. 3.41: Bruise over upper end tibia

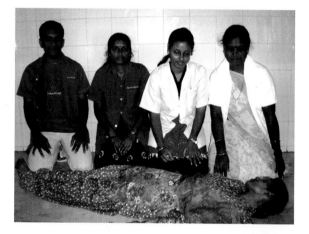

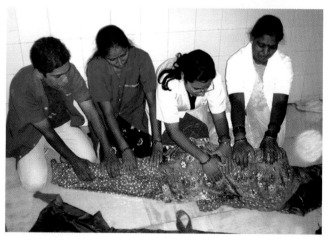

Fig. 4.2 (Contd.)

Plate 3

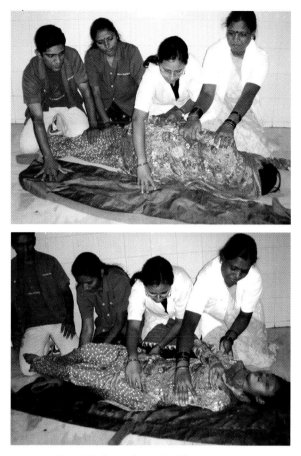

Fig. 4.2: Logroll method for transport

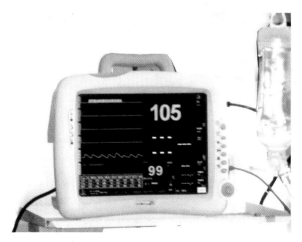

Fig. 4.3: Monitor

Plate 4

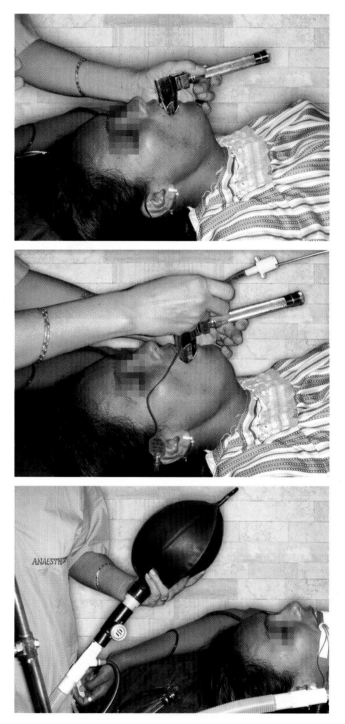

Fig. 4.11: Steps of intubation

CHAPTER 1

General Principles of Trauma Management

Introduction

What is Trauma?

Trauma is unavoidable incident or damage occurring suddenly to living part, that is beyond body's resilience.

In 2010, road trauma ranked 6th as cause of death in world table.

In 2020 it is estimated to be in 3rd place.

Today every one person dies in every six minutes on Indian roads.

By 2020, rate is expected to be more than one in every 3 minutes.

According to the Indian injury report 2010, injury is the 3rd cause of mortality in India.

Perhaps for this reason trauma is moving up the political agenda as one of only four themes in UK government's latest strategy of "Our Healthier Nation".

High velocity trauma is number one cause of death in 18 to 44 years of age group world wide.

In US, loss of income due to death and disability resulting from high velocity trauma totals more than 75 billions dollar annually-huge economic loss to the government.

Goal of all governmental agencies is to minimize mortality and maximize return in this economically productive segment of population.

Despite of these major economic productive losses, less than 2% of total research budget is given in US.

So, for funding of research in injury prevention and trauma management, legislation must be passed, designed to minimize morbidity and mortality from vehicular accident.

History

History is a bowl of spaghetti, with all the strands being entangled together. Writing about history is like lifting up one strand and trying to find the end without having it to break (Fig. 1.1).

History gives us the opportunity to see the natural evolution of disease.

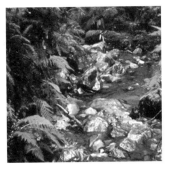

Fig. 1.1: Story of creativity

History of trauma dates back to ancient times in 3500 BC, where surgeons of ancient Egypt dressed wound, performing amputation and removing foreign body.

In the 5th century Hippocrates, the Greeks described fracture, dislocations and wounds.

Modern principles of acute trauma care begins in 20th century.

Today, we are treating disease early and have lost the day-to-day familiarity with its untreated course that physician formerly required.

Transformation to its current form has been achieved by prevention more than by treatment.

How Trauma Management Evolves?

"History is a story of *creativity.*"

About 500 years ago,

Trauma **began in jungles**, (Fig. 1.2) our foresfathers with bow and arrow, archery, protected themselves from wild animals, injuries were not much serious, and treated with local herbs and ayurveda techniques, splinting fractures with tree branches.

Later comes an **era of wars** (Fig. 1.3) with sword, bow and arrow, human being started fighting with each other for survival. During World War I and II come gunshot injuries, which still continue, injuries were crucial, but life saving. Knowledge of first aid, blood transfusion, wound dressing, along with medical and ayurveda came into existence.

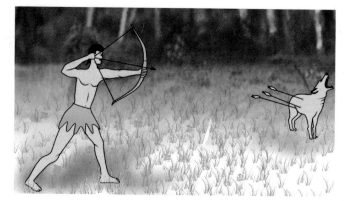

Fig. 1.2: Hunting in the jungle

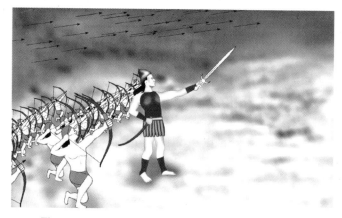

Fig. 1.3: An era of wars with sword, bow and arrow

After 1960, (Fig. 1.4) **an era of industrial revolution** began all over world and machine injuries came into action, these were serious but life saving injuries. Concept of prevention of disability with reconstructive surgeries began and medical revolution of surgery and its tactics also began in this era.

Presently, we are living in era of *21st century where* everything is instant, it's an **era of automobile** (Fig. 1.5), *it is not life saving, it is life-threatening injuries.* This is the most recent advances in field of medicine with concept of resuscitation, ABC of management.

Thereby **'Golden Hour'** treatment comes into existence.

> "History is a story of stupid mistakes."

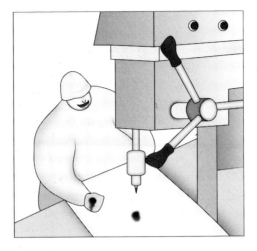

Fig. 1.4: An era of machine injury

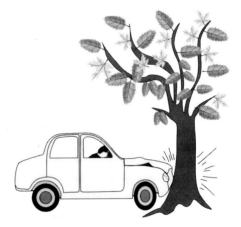

Fig. 1.5: An era of automobile injury

 Today, car and pedestrian injuries provide most serious trauma in particularly developing countries.

Ironically, Nicholas-Joseph Cugnot (1725 –1804), a French army captain, who invented (1770) the first automobile was injured by it.

"History is evidence for evidence based behavior."

How Advanced Trauma Life Support (ATLS) Developed?

Advanced trauma life support (ATLS) is trauma management guidelines published by American

College of Surgeons and provide frame work for the management of injured person.

The ATLS has its origin in the US in 1976, when an orthopedic surgeon, piloting a light aircraft, crashed his plane into a field in Nebraska. His wife was killed instantly and three of his four children received critical injuries.

He was appalled enough at the haphazard treatment of his children, so he was to change the face of trauma cases throughout the world. Various medical, EMS and nursing groups within Nebraska region began a set of protocol for the management of trauma patient, these were then taken up and modified by the American College of Surgeons and published a ATLS in 1980.

Dr Sejal's Principles of Trauma Management

- Timely aggressive involvement of person during 'golden hour' of trauma management.
- Definitive protocols of detail management with productive working of trauma care system.
- Accurate assessment, action and management results in early and quick recovery.
- Proper understanding of anatomical and physiological changes in particular trauma results in good outcome.

Dr Sejal's Classification of Trauma Management

Management of trauma begins from event and site itself and it ends till body starts functioning physiologically and anatomically.

Management According to

Time

- Early at site
- Late at tertiary center
- Delayed after twenty-four hours.

Difference in different age group

- Pediatric
- Adult
- Geriatric

Severity of injury

- Life-threatening
- Life-saving

Anatomical parts

- Head, neck, chest, abdomen, limbs....

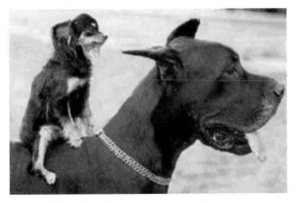

Goals of Trauma Management

- To save life with minimum disability
- It should be available to each and every injured person at any time and any place.
- Deficiency in resources and organization should be overcome.
- To bring out patient from site with spinal precaution and transport patient immediately to medical center.
- Early fast look over pulse—vitals, bleeding, consciousness, cause of trauma.
- Start treatment with whatever available like stick, pints, and clothes for bleeding, liquids/juices for diabetics.
- Early proper rehabilitation can change the outcome.

  "Normally there are three stages of illness (trauma)
  1st – ill
  2nd – pill
  3rd – bill and sometimes the 4th stage – will
  We don't want this 4th stage in action."

Fig. 1.6: Always help a friend in need

Knowledge of management of trauma is the first help at any place, in any circumstances and with anybody, so doctors, paramedics and even a layman must have it.

Act and Avoid Fear Factor

Do's and Don'ts in Trauma Management

Do's	Don'ts
• Be calm	• Do not be panic
• Act fast	• Do not waste time
• Be strong	• Don't be afraid of medico-legal problems
• Make fast decision	• Don't dither or wait till doctor or expert arrives
• Ask for help	• Don't discuss/argue with anybody
• Help yourself	• Don't wait for help
• Act it	• Don't react it

Any situation can worsen by getting panic

- As ones mind gets paralyzed.
- One can take wrong judgment.
- Even a small mistake can convert problem into tragedy.
- At the end, one will lose something (patient/ credit/ both).

You don't have time to stumble, fumble or forget

So,

Let your first aid be best aid

In trauma to diagnose disease is easy as compared to other branches but to treat and manage patient is very, very difficult. So if you manage trauma properly, there is least chances of morbidity and impairment to many lives.

90% of traumas are man made trauma, only 10% traumas are uncontrollable nature's gift.

"So trauma evolves from ourselves and treated by ourselves and ends with ourselves".

So be kind, good, and courageous to your fellow beings and protect God's gift, never overcome it or you have to lose lives and ourselves.

Criteria to Face Emergencies

- You should be mentally, physically fit.
- You should be very sound in your basic knowledge of emergency.
- You should be good and remember your ethics.
- You should be well versed with the procedure and trained properly.

    Legislation should be passed to make compulsory study for children in school, adults in colleges, offices, factories, all government institutions as a mandatory functional curriculum for basic trauma management.

> Treat   Life   Before   Limbs

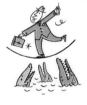

Pitfall in Trauma Management

- Lack of knowledge/education of trainee/ person/ society
- Lack of infrastructure
- Lack of government support
- Lack of training/educational centers, continuous medical education, and awareness programs.
- Lack of guidance for proper usage of machines, procedures.
- Lack of strict follow-up of laws.

Recent Advances in Trauma Management

- *"Damage control"* has become standard care to seriously injured patient rather than providing definitive treatment for all of the injured patient.
- One of the goal of resuscitation is identification and control of life-threatening hemorrhage.

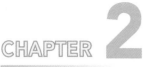

CHAPTER 2

Trauma Care System

What is Trauma Care System?

A trauma care system is an organized, coordinated, well-managed effort in given or defined geographic area that delivers the full range of trauma care to all injured patients with the help of local and public health system.

Aim of Trauma Care System

- Reduction of injury incidence and its severity.
- Rigorous (arrange something in order to get maximum advantage) system performance.
- Cost containment and efficacy enhancement.

Function of Trauma Care System

- Set objectives
- Develop action plan
- Conduct tactical operation
- Provide logistics support
- Financial provision and accounting.

Model of Trauma Care System

As soon as a call or information regarding happening or accident is received, nearby **Prehospital trauma team** approaches to site, *During transport* ambulance crew member continue with ABC's, detailing of patient with history, age, address, past medical history (Fig. 2.1).

Once ambulance reaches the hospital, **Hospital trauma team** takes over the function. On receiving patient to hospital, patient status during enroute is notified to examining doctor.

The ambulance crew should wait to see if the receiving trauma physician has any question about prior treatment or conditions on the accident scene. He/she should left only thereafter with permission of trauma captain.

Dr Sejal's Trauma Care System

Thus trauma care system is divided into:
- Prehospital trauma care system
- Hospital trauma care system.

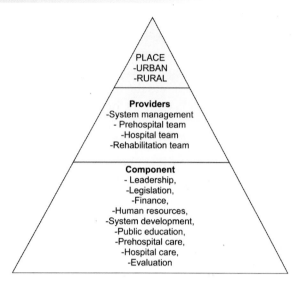

Fig. 2.1: A model of trauma care system

Prehospital and Hospital Trauma Care System

Tenon called hospitals "machines for health."

Hospitals were originally places for the poor to die.

When a patient shows signs of recovery from any condition another fatal condition took its place.

In the past, people used to go to the hospital at the end of a disease—now they go at the beginning.

Team of Prehospital and Hospital Trauma Care System Includes

Prehospital Team	Hospital Team

• Ambulance crew members like
  – EMT's (emergency medical technician)
  – nurses
  – compatible ambulance driver
• Nonmedical person
• Community workers
• Health providers
• Government bodies like police, army
• Aid and relief agencies.
	• Captain
	• Senior trauma surgeon
	• Trauma consultant
	• Surgical house staff
	• Anesthesiologist
	• Radio technician
	• CT technician
	• Operating room staff
	• Nursing team
	• Trauma physician
	• Administrative personnel.

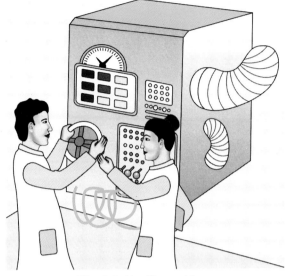

Fig. 2.2: Health machines

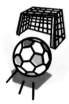

Goals of Prehospital and Hospital Trauma Care System

In 19th century, there was a rise in status, power and wealth of doctor.

They organized and took up technology. Physician, surgeon, orthopedician came closure and shared knowledge, set common goals, criteria and critical role

Prehospital Goals	Hospital Goals
• Efficient and sustainable approach • Rescue • Stabilization • Transport of patient	• To save life • Smooth efficient, result oriented outcome • Discharge patient with minimum or no disability.

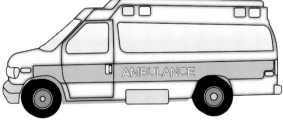

Fig. 2.3: Ambulance

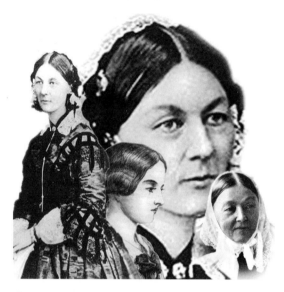

Fig. 2.4: Florence Nightingale

of team members to improve the prognosis of the patient and management of hospital, with trauma management.

Criteria for Prehospital and Hospital Trauma Care System

"The Lady with the Lamp", Florence Nightingale founded the concept of modern nursing. Her criteria are very useful in management of mass casualities and in disaster management.

Prehospital Criteria	Hospital Criteria

• Universal toll free health line/ communicating devices accessible and easily available, user friendly.
 • Ambulance well equipped
 • Support from health worker, community worker, EMT's and government bodies for smooth running of system.
 • Proper triage—no under/over triage during mass causalities and disasters.
 • Easy, advanced mode of transportation—air, water, land.
	• Efficient surgeon or trauma physician and team
	  – 24 × 7 availability
	  – Experience
	  – Aggressiveness
	  – Daring
	  – Flexibility
	  – Courage
	  – Decisiveness
	  – Knowledge.
	 • Advanced life management
	  – Equipments
	  – Laboratory
	  – Blood bank facility
	  – Well-equipped operation theater and ICU
	  – All specialty and subspecialty back up.
	 • Advanced rehabilitation unit

Critical Role in Prehospital and Hospital Trauma Care Management

Critical Role in Prehospital	Critical Role in Hospital

Critical Role in Prehospital

- Dedicated medical director
- Prehospital trauma team is governed by communicating device to final decision maker- The Team captain.
- Effective transport
- Well trained EMT in specific intervention
- Team members help to remove patient from site,
- Rapid assessment of the patient with quick history and cause of trauma,
- Give first aid.
- Helps ambulance crew to continue treatment and transport.

Critical Role in Hospital

- Trauma captain,
- Familiar with team members' skills and capabilities to do the work, facilitating optimal outcome.
- Evaluation and management of day to day injured cases.
- Maintenance of records. Guide and coordinate activities of team members.
- Make critical treatment and triage decision.

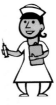

Trauma nurse coordinator
- Monitors the progress of the patient.
- Particular attention to prevent complication of injury.
- Helps and assists the team.

- Trauma registry
- To review trends in management outcome.
- To measure performance of the system and to change clinical care to improve patient's recovery from injury.
- Group meeting on monthly basis for discussion of problems, review of poor outcome, dissemination and development of new protocols, improvement of rapport.
- Medical records for research work.

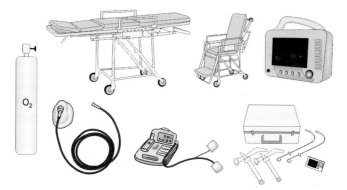

Fig. 2.5: Ambulance with necessary equipment

What are Requirements in Emergency Room?

- Fowler bed
- Crash trolley
- Intubation set
- Ventilator functioning
- Oxygen uninterrupted
- Dressing tray
- Monitors hi-tech
- Syringe pump
- Procedure room
- On call doctors list
- Working telephone or communicating devices
- Prohibited area
- Clean fumigated, sterile room.

How to Protect Trauma Team?

Trauma team member should be protected by disease.

All Trauma team members are to wear PPE (Fig. 2.8) (Personal Protection Equipment) such as:

- Gloves
- Waterproof apron/gowns
- Mask
- Protective eyewear

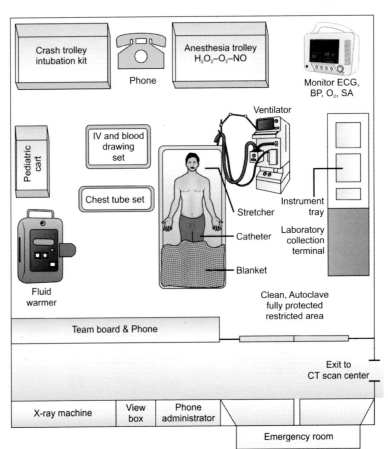

Fig. 2.6: Trauma room organization

 ## Disaster Management

Disaster occurs without knocking at the door and so its planning is an essential part to any trauma management. A simple disaster planning includes

- Disaster scenarios practice
- Disaster management protocols
  - On scene management
  - Key personnel identification
  - Trauma triage
  - Medical team allocation from the hospital
  - Aggrement in advance on who will be involved in the event of a disaster.
    — Ambulance
    — Police/army

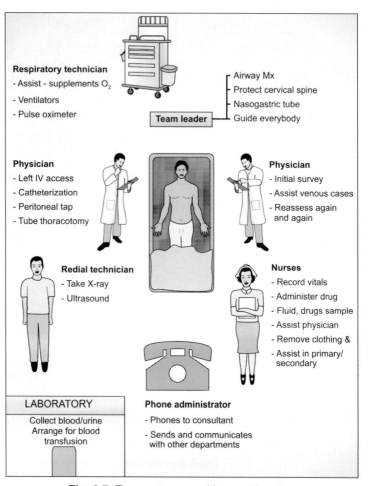

Respiratory technician
- Assist - supplements O_2
- Ventilators
- Pulse oximeter

- Airway Mx
- Protect cervical spine
- Nasogastric tube
- Guide everybody

Team leader

Physician
- Left IV access
- Catheterization
- Peritoneal tap
- Tube thoracotomy

Physician
- Initial survey
- Assist venous cases
- Reassess again and again

Redial technician
- Take X-ray
- Ultrasound

Nurses
- Record vitals
- Administer drug
- Fluid, drugs sample
- Assist physician
- Remove clothing &
- Assist in primary/ secondary

LABORATORY

Collect blood/urine
Arrange for blood transfusion

Phone administrator
- Phones to consultant
- Sends and communicates with other departments

Fig. 2.7: Trauma team position and function

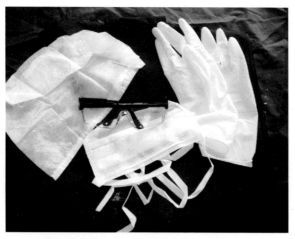

Fig. 2.8: Personal protection equipment

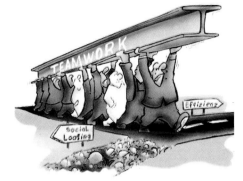

Fig. 2.9: Work together as a team *(Courtesy: Google image)*

- — National and international authorities
- — Aid and relief agencies and media
- – Evacuation priorities
- – Modes of transport – road/air/sea.
- – Communication strategies.

"Prevention is wholesale and treatment is retail."

Triage

It is pronounced *(tree-ahz)* a French word used to indicate sorting and classification of injured and establishment of treatment, priorities in situation like mass causalities as earth quake, bus/train accident, natural calamities.

What is Triage?

Triage is disciplinized screening and classi-fication of severely wounded and injured persons during war, mass casualties, disaster, and natural calamities to determine priority needs for efficient use of doctor, nurse and paramedics staff in emergency room or else where.

"A stitch in time saves nine."

Historically

It is an old concept since war time, when soldiers more injured were snatched or took off from battlefield and were transported to emergency care away from battlefield.

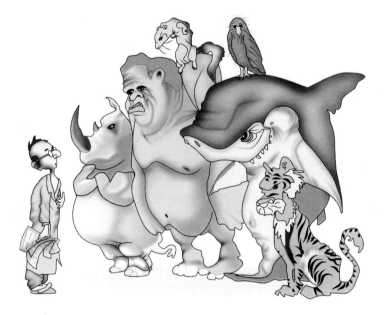

Fig. 2.10: Sorting out danger one first

Triage is one part of paramedical management of trauma. It is just like planning your business, or finance.

Advantage and Importance of Triage

- It saves maximum number of lives.
- Smooth hassle free running of emergencies
- Avoids chaos, anxiety
- Avoids unnecessary over treatment to less wounded and necessary life saving treatment to more wounded persons.
- Helps better, early transport to emergency room with prompt treatment.

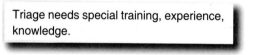

Triage needs special training, experience, knowledge.

Triage itself starts from the site of disaster, accident or battle field.

Who can be Involved in Triage?

Doctors, nurse, paramedics, layman, admini-strative personality or available anybody can participate.

The captain – reaches site, if possible and quickly understands situation in seconds/ minutes and acts fast accordingly.

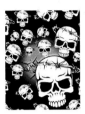

Triage Screens out Most Wounded—How?

With the help of nurse or paramedic in few seconds
- Brief history
- Vitals
- Rapid physical examination
- Perform first aid
- ABC's of triage
- Reassessment according to severity
- Transport to emergency room or appropriate place.

Before approaching to patient,
Look for,
- *Vehicle is stable, will it roll or move.*
- *Split fuel*
- *Risk of fire*
- *Any power poles involved*
- *What about out coming traffic?*

> Do not touch anything until you are sure that it is safe to touch.

Control the road traffic accident scene by asking bystander to:
- Redirect traffic
- Asking children and adult to move back.
- Not to smoke near site or damaged vehicle.

Parameters in Triage
- Neurological
- Respiratory
- Perfusion.

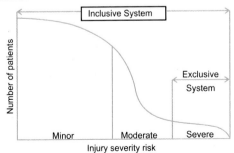

Fig. 2.11

Over Triage (Fig. 2.12)

Occurs, when noncritical patients are sent to facilities offering the highest level of care.

Under Triage (Fig. 2.13)

Occurs, when critically injured patients are neglected or treated at the local level or sent to facilities that are not properly equipped to meet their needs. This can result in increase in morbidity and mortality.

This basics of triage each and every medical personnel, nurse, paramedics must know.

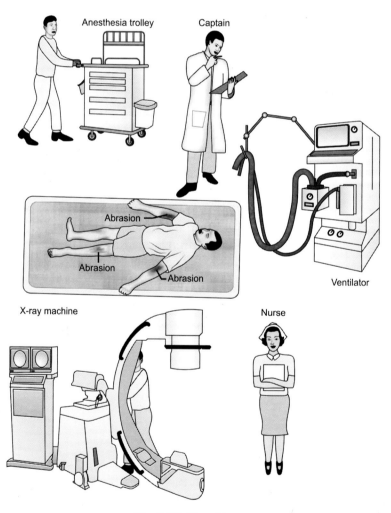

Fig. 2.12: Over triage

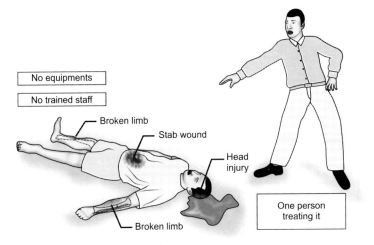

Fig. 2.13: Under triage

"Your inefficient knowledge can sink titanic of lives of many."

Effective triage can satisfy you, patient, governing media, body or government.

Pitfalls in Triage
- Less paramedical staff
- Fewer personnel
- Lack or no knowledge to staff/personnel

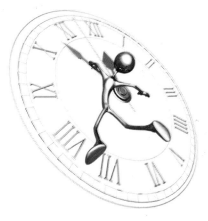

Fig. 2.14: Golden hour of trauma management

- No mode of transportation/communication. In such situation, ask for help from outside. Don't feel shy because triage is a team work.

> Triage is a part of 'golden hours' in emergency trauma management, so don't waste it.

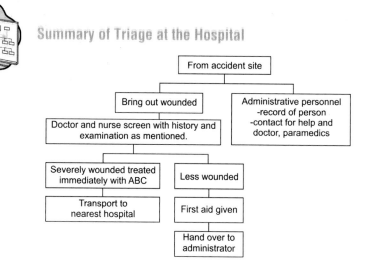

Summary of Triage at the Hospital

```
                    From accident site
              ┌──────────┴──────────┐
      Bring out wounded      Administrative personnel
                              -record of person
  Doctor and nurse screen     -contact for help and
  with history and            doctor, paramedics
  examination as mentioned.
        ┌─────────┴─────────┐
  Severely wounded treated   Less wounded
  immediately with ABC
        │                        │
   Transport to            First aid given
   nearest hospital             │
                          Hand over to
                          administrator
```

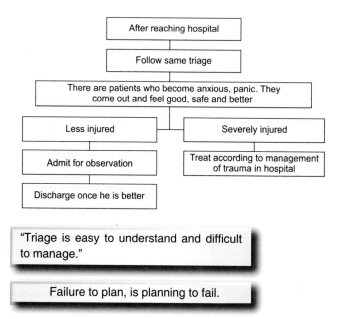

Summary of Triage at the Hospital

```
              After reaching hospital
                       │
             Follow same triage
                       │
  There are patients who become anxious, panic. They
        come out and feel good, safe and better
        ┌──────────────┴──────────────┐
   Less injured                 Severely injured
        │                            │
  Admit for observation      Treat according to management
        │                    of trauma in hospital
  Discharge once he is better
```

> "Triage is easy to understand and difficult to manage."

> Failure to plan, is planning to fail.

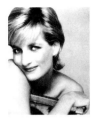

A Story of Princess of Wales " Diana"

It was Saturday 30th August 1997, Diana and Dodi's holidays came to an end. They still wanted to spend some more time. They landed in Paris in the afternoon. They were followed by photographers. They stayed in Al-Fayed Villa and dined at Ritz hotel. The photographers still following them, they wanted to have some good snaps of the couple. At Ritz, evasive action taken by Dodi with the help of hotel staff, Mr Henry Paul, a security person. At 19 minutes past midnight, Diana and Dodi asked Henry to drive the car with their bodyguard from back exit.

But paparazzi still followed them and soon there were many photographers. Henry Paul wanted to ovedrive them. He drove faster and faster and raced them into the tunnel. The speed limit was 80 km and he drove at 180 km. Shortly after entrance car skid, lurched from side to side and exploded with 13th concrete post. It was 00:25 minutes. The driver and Dodi lost their life on scene. Bodyguard sitting on front seat with belt was unconscious but alive. Lady Diana was breathing. By chance, on opposite carriage way a doctor was driving, he saw the car accident and stopped his car. He saw Diana make rowing movement with her arms, when injured people do this, it means they are not receiving oxygen. He gave oxygen with mask, the ambulance was underway. It took almost one hour until she was taken out of wreck by cutting metal sheats and reached hospital.

At half past one in the morning, Diana came into the hospital's emergency operation theater. The surgeons opened her rib cage and discovered torn vein. Massive inner bleeding present. They managed to control it. But, suddenly heart stopped. They tried to bring back the life of the princess by cardiac massage. The fight lasted till morning 4 o'clock and the doctors had to agree that they had lost the fight.

Diana was dead!

The princess of Wales died on 31st August 1997 at 3.57 am.

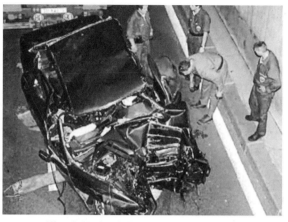

Fig. 2.15: Lady Diana's car accident

Many things to learn:
- Henry Paul was drunk
- Driving beyond speed limit
- No seat belts worn by Diana and Dodi
- It took authority long time to make her reach the hospital – thus GOLDEN HOURS were lost.

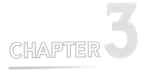

Trauma Management at Site

- When to Do Cardiopulmonary Resuscitation?
- Goals of Cardiopulmonary Resuscitation.
- How to give Chest Compression?
- Infant Cardiopulmonary Resuscitation
  - How to know Partial Obstruction?
  - How to give Cardiopulmonary Resuscitation?
  - When to stop Cardiopulmonary Resuscitation?
- Recent advances in Cardiopulmonary Resuscitation
- How to Manage Bleeding at Site?
- ○ Disability
  - How to Manage Head Injury at Site?
- ○ Exposure.
- ➲ Secondary Survey
  - ○ Chest Injury—First Aid Tricks
  - ○ Abdominal Injury
  - ○ Pelvic Injury
  - ○ Spine Injury
  - ○ Fracture
    - How to Diagnose It?
    - How to Manage Fracture at Site?
    - How to know Bandage is Tight?
    - How to Treat Tight Bandage?
  - ○ Crush Injury
    - What to Look for?
    - How to Treat Initially?
- ➲ Preparation for Transport

Once you know the principles and trauma care system is working, your journey to management begins.

When you find yourself in this situation how to manage such patient?

Begin with

First Aid

Definition

It is the initial assistance or care of a suddenly injured person.

It is important part of everyday life at home, work, or play.

Everybody should learn first aid and be willing to administer basic prompt care and attention prior to the arrival of the ambulance or assistance, this can sometimes mean the differences between the life and death or between full or partial recovery.

Aim

- To preserve the life
- To protect the injured from further harm.
- To provide pain relief—applying sling, splint or icepacks, etc.
- To give reassurance

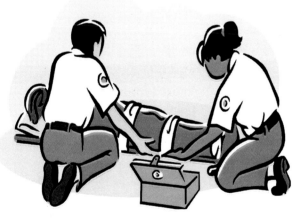

Fig. 3.1: EMT's with first aid box

> Immediate action is the essential principle of first aid.

How to React?

- Call for help.
- Don't be panic.
- Recognize the basic symptoms of injury.
- Plan action.
- Remain cool and calm and think your action thoroughly, it will give you confidence and will handle event efficient and effectively.

  Each emergency is different, so it is impossible to provide with a precise list of things you need to do for every emergency.

What should be there in First Aid Kit?

- Band aids
- Adhesive tapes
- Alcohol swabs
- Gauze swabs
- Disposable gloves
- Nonadhesive dressings
- Plastic bags for amputates
- Safety pins
- Dressing pad-sterile
- Crepe bandage
- Scissors
- Triangular bandage.

Primary Survey

What should be Done?

- Never leave injured at site of accident. First rescue injured from the site of accident by yourself or with help of others.
- Identify whether injured is conscious or drowsy or talking—this will give you idea whether airway, breathing is patent or not?
- Don't miss to look for pulse preferably femoral or jugular (Fig. 3.2).
- Start ABC's with spinal precaution.

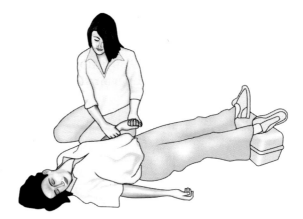

Fig. 3.2: Checking pulse and elevation of leg

Basic Trauma Life Support

What is Basic Trauma Life Support?

Cardiopulmonary resuscitation is a combination of rescue breathing and chest compression which forms basic trauma life support.

An ultra quick diagnostic assessment within 10 to 15 seconds.

What are Prerequisites before Initiating Basic Trauma Life Support?

- To call for help
- To give appropriate position of victim
- To give appropriate position of rescuer.

Basic life support
Precordial thump
Clear airway
Maintain ventilation by mouth to mouth respiration
Maintain circulation by external chest compression
Proceed to advanced life support

Fig. 3.3: Flow chat for basic trauma life support

Airway

To check whether obstructed or not (Fig. 3.4)

To clear the obstruction from mouth till upper trachea and allow proper air ventilation and tissue oxygenation to body.

Obstruction can be
- Blood
- Mucus
- Clot
- Saliva
- Fractures
- Injury to trachea

How to know Airway Obstruction?
- Snoring or gurgling
- Stridor
- Abnormal breath
- Hypoxia
- Using accessory muscles for ventilation or paradoxical chest movement, cyanosis
- Be aware of foreign body.

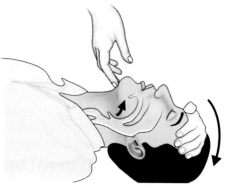

Normal airway

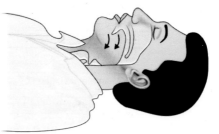

Obstructed airway open in neutral position

Fig. 3.4: Normal airway like this

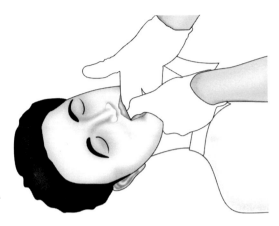

Fig. 3.5: Removing visible debris from mouth

How to remove visible obstruction? (Fig. 3.5)

Remove it by opening the mouth and inserting finger as shown with spinal precaution.

Breathing

How to Check Breathing Adequacy?

Look, listen, feel.

Once airway patency is assessed (Fig. 3.6)
* Look-chest risse, retraction, nasal flares.
* Listen—to breath sounds, stridor and obstructed ventilation.
* Feel—air inhale and exhale against your finger/ check.

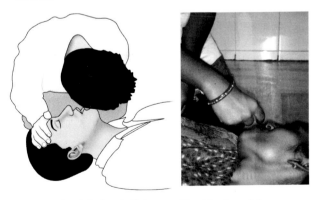

Fig. 3.6: Look, listen and feel for breathing
(*For color version, see Plate 1*)

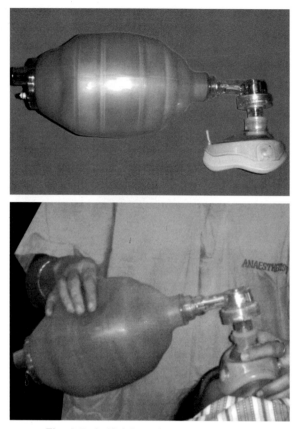

Fig. 3.7: Artificial ventilation (Ambu Bag)
(*For color version, see Plate 1*)

Airway Management

- Check airway patency by talking to patient, if patient speaks/talks clearly must have clear airway. Airway obstruction by tongue in the unconscious patient is often a problem, the unconscious patient may require assistance with airway and ventilation.
- Assess the airway, if mild obstruction- encourage coughing.
- Give oxygen, if available via self-inflating bag or mask.

Method

- Position of patient—hard surface or neutral head.
- Position of rescuer—kneel on side of patient.
- Ensure open airway and place your hand on forehead.

- Place your other fingertips under the injured chin and gently tilt the head back and lift the chin to open the airway.

Tip

> Never mistaken head position with neck extension.

- Remove visible foreign body, all debris, clots, blood with the help of handkerchief or gauze piece with finger.
  Two types of head tilt in resuscitation:
- Neutral—used for infants and suspected spinal injury
- Backward—older children, adult, elderly

Tip

> - Do not give excessive forces especially if injury to neck is suspected.
> - In children, do not press on the soft tissue under chin as this may block airway further.

Once the airway is maintained, vomiting of stomach contents, tongue fall, fluid, or other object and inhalation cause obstruction.

> Ensure and check regularly for tongue fall, it may further obstruct airway.

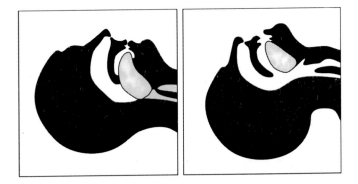

Fig. 3.8: Tongue blocking airways

Trick

> To keep injured in lateral or recovery position with spinal precaution on the same side with head down and tilted in such a way that vomit expels and tongue doesn't fall and clear the airway.

If injured is to be kept in recovery position for maximum 30 minutes, it is advisable to turn them over to other side.

How to Give Back Blow? (Figs 3.9 and 3.10)

- Position yourself to deliver back blows—slightly behind to the side of injured.
- Lean injured well forward.
- Support chest from front with one hand.
- Deliver five firm back blows between shoulder blades using heel of hand.

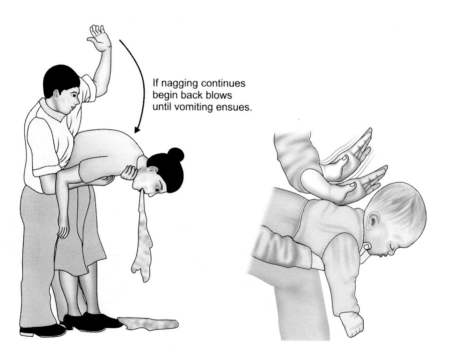

If nagging continues begin back blows until vomiting ensues.

Fig. 3.9: Back blows in adult **Fig. 3.10:** Back blows in children

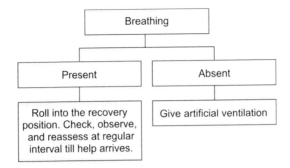

Fig. 3.11: Flow chart for breathing

- Check mouth and clear after each back blow.
- Repeat till obstruction is relieved.
- If obstruction is at the entrance to trachea, slap may cause the person to inhale the object and cause complete obstruction.

Tip

Do not slap them on back.

If you are in any doubt that the injured is breathing normally, treat as if they are not breathing.

Artificial Ventilation

Breath for the person.

Rescue breaths

Rescue breathing is in fact breathing for *unconscious* person, who is having pulse but is not breathing. It's effective method of buying time.

Rescue breath = mouth to mouth resuscitation

Five main methods for delivering rescue breaths:

Mouth to Mouth resuscitation

Position—Use head tilt and a chin lift to keep victim's airway open as mentioned (Fig. 3.12).

Method—
- Pinch the nose, rescuer seals the injured mouth with his own mouth and then blows air into the injured mouth. Pause in between each breath to let the air flow out.

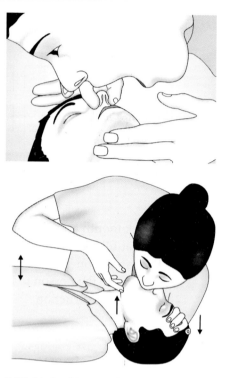

Fig. 3.12: Method for mouth to mouth resuscitation

- Look for chest rise and fall, if not, retilt and try again.
- If air still does not go in—look for airway obstructed and perform abdominal thrusts.
- Give 1 breath every 5 seconds.

Mouth to nose

Used in facial injury

Rescuer covers the nose with his mouth, breaths gently and releases the injured jaw to allow exhalation.

Mouth to nose and mouth

Used for resuscitating an infant or young children, a rescuer mouth covers and seals the mouth and nose of infant.

Mouth to mask

It is the recent and most desirable method, as the risk of cross infection is lessened compared to mouth to mouth.

Brook Mask, 'S' shape mask is fitted firmly over the nose and mouth and rescuer delivers rescue breaths via the valve or tube thus avoiding direct contact with injured mouth.

Rescue breaths are considered effective only, if the chest rise and falls with each breath.

For infants

- The method used is "frog breathing" or "puffy". Where rescuer fills his/her mouth with air and "Puffs" into the infant's mouth.
- There will be adequate pressure and volume to satisfy lung requirements.
- To open the airway of an infant or child, you do not need to tilt the head as that of an adults. A very slight tilt should allow air to go in (Fig. 3.13 step 1).
- Give 1 slow breath every 3 second, after one minute check for a pulse.
- If breaths still do not go in, you must go immediately to abdominal thrusts.
- If air delivered too forceful, it will be directed in stomach and forced to cause vomit, obstructing further airway.

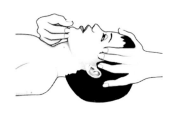

Step 1   Step 2

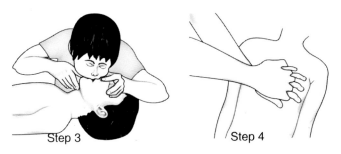

Step 3   Step 4

Fig. 3.13: Children airway above 5 years

When to stop giving rescue breaths?

Only when

- The injured begins to breath on his/her own.
- The injured has no pulse – begin CPR immediately.
- Advanced medical help arrives or takes over.
- You are physically too exhausted to continue.

Circulation

Loss of circulation to any vital organ can cause disturbance to organ, leading to failure and death of an organ.

Circulation can be achieved in case of sudden cardiac arrest by precordial thump as first line of treatment.

Precordial thump (commonly seen in drama-Hindi movies) (Fig. 3.14).

- Indication—Initially during cardiac arrest, when no defibrillator available.
- Needs proper training.
- Used only when arrest is monitored (by pulse, palpable heart sound).
- Should be used only once during cardiac arrest.
- **Method**—One or two forceful blows with fist are delivered from a height of 8 to 10 inches roughly at junction of middle and lower third of sternum. Such

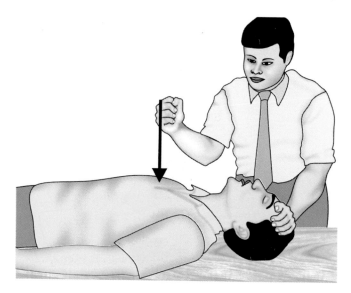

Fig. 3.14: Chest thump

thump delivers a low level of electric depolarization current of approx 2 to 5 joules.
- Adverse effect—Additional injuries to chest and lung are noted.

How to Give Cardiac Massage?

Perhaps most frightening thing for a rescue worker is to have a victim's heart stop.

If injured is not breathing and no pulse is there, start with CPR.

Why to do CPR?

- Cardiopulmonary resuscitation (CPR) helps to restore circulation of oxygen rich blood to the brain.
- Helps to restore normal physiology and function of an organ.

When to do CPR?

- Cardiopulmonary resuscitation may be necessary during many different emergencies, accident, drowning, suffocation, poisoning, smoke inhalation.
- Unconscious
- No normal breathing.

Goals of CPR

In most of uncomplicated cases the goals of resuscitation are:
- To increase
  - Blood pressure
  - Urine output
  - Capillary perfusion
  - Conscious level
  - Oxygen saturation.
- To decrease
  - Heart rate

CPR can be done by two techniques:
- Single person technique
- Two person technique.

Single Person Technique

- Position of injured and rescuer as mentioned.
- Open airway.
- Blow gush of air into victim's mouth for about one second.

- Give chest compression as mentioned.
- Give second breath.
- Continue this cycle till pulse is present or help arrives, if no pulse present, continue CPR.
- If pulse is present but no breathing, go for rescue breathing.

How to give Chest Compression?

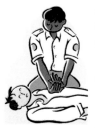

- Kneel by patient side.
- Find the tip of xiphoid process of sternum and palpate lower chest.
- Place heel of one hand in the center of injured chest, next place heel of the other hand on top of first hand and interlock the fingers of the hands (Fig. 3.18).
- With arm straight and position yourself directly on the sternum, your shoulder should be directly over your hands, press down 1/3 depth of chest.
- Compression at a rate of about 100 times / min.

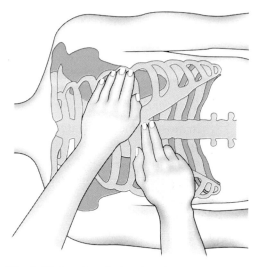

Fig. 3.15: Landmarks to give chest compression

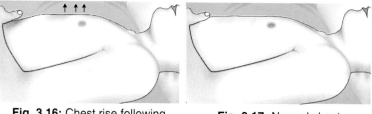

Fig. 3.16: Chest rise following each CPR

Fig. 3.17: Normal chest

Remember

If you push directly down on xiphoid or lower chest, you will likely to rupture the injured liver and perhaps few other vital organs and all the CPR in the world are helpless.

Don't forget

Keep synchronization by giving two breaths with each 15 compressions.

Tip

Fix chin and head, closed nostril before you blow gush of air over patient mouth.
Look for chest rise with each breath.

Two-Person Technique
- First person does mouth respiration.
- Second person does chest compression.
- Compression and release should take an equal time, count a loud "one, two and three…", etc. as you do the compressions, maintaining a smooth, steady rhythm (Fig. 3.19).

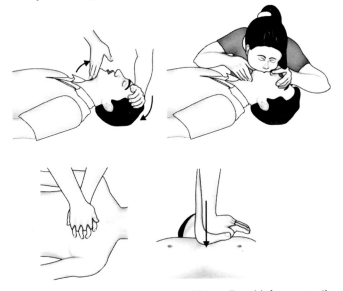

Fig. 3.18: Single person technique with handkerchief over mouth and nose close with finger and giving blow with mouth as shown in photo.

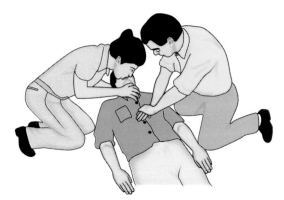

Fig. 3.19: Two-person technique

- Recheck for sign of life while continuing compression.
  If rescue breath do not make the chest rise with each attempt proceed 15 compressions, if it failed
- Check the victim's mouth and remove visible obstruction.
- Ensure also adequate head tilt and chin lift.
  If for any reason rescue breaths cannot be given or failed, continue chest compression, as some of oxygen will still be circulated.

> Do not attempt more than two rescue breaths each time before returning to chest compression.

Infants CPR

How to know partial obstruction in children?

- Flaring of the nostrils.
- In drawing of the tissue above the sternum and between the ribs.

How to give CPR in children or infant?

- Kneel by side
- Draw an imaginary line across the infant's chest between the infant's nipples.
- Place your index finger on sternum just below this imaginary line in the center of infant's chest (Fig. 3.20).
- Position yourself above the chest with the two-finger, compress the chest ½ to 1 inch.

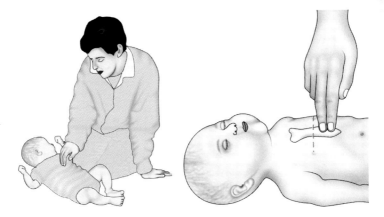

Fig. 3.20: Infant CPR two-finger technique

- Release all pressure on the chest without losing contact between fingers and sternum.
- Compression and release should take an equal amount of time.
- Be sure to do a very slight head tilt and chin lift to open the airway when giving breaths.
- Give five chest compressions and one breath. After one minute of continuous CPR (about 12 cycles), check for brachial pulse.
- If pulse is present, but no breath, continue rescue breath.
- Continue it till pulse and breath present or help arrives.

Tip

Never use hand, use finger only and give firm equal pressure and release.

When to stop CPR?

- Victim starts breath and pulse present.
- More advanced medical help arrives and take over.
- You are too exhausted and become physically unable to continue.

Recent Advances in CPR

- Alternative method to CPR is CCR (Cardio- cerebral resuscitation) which is under trial claims 300% greater success rate over standard CPR.

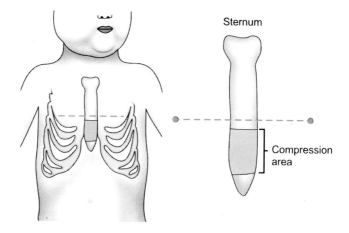

Sternum

Compression area

Fig. 3.21: Landmarks for infant CPR

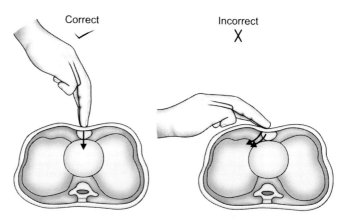

Correct

Incorrect

Fig. 3.22: Chest compression

- Exceptions are in case of drowning or drug overdose.
- Rhythmic abdominal compression works by forcing blood from blood vessels around the abdominal organs known to contain 25% of the body's total blood volume. This blood is redirected to other sites, including the circulation around the heart.
- **Advantage**—To avoid mouth to mouth breathing and eliminate the risk of rib fracture and transfer of infection.

Remember

> Any resuscitation is better than no resuscitation at all.

Resuscitation attempts after 10 to 15 minutes of arrest have rarely been found to be successful.

How to manage bleeding at site?

Once CPR is achieved and patient is stable or unstable, along with look for type of bleeding (arterial, venous, oozing).

Loss of blood can be
- External/visible
- Internal/invisible

Basic tips in controlling of bleeding:

External *visible* loss can be controlled by

Apply RED

- Rest—it will decrease heart rate
- Elevate—injured site above the level of heart in order to reduce blood loss at the site.
- Direct pressure—over wound with sterile dressing and apply a firm bandage to hold dressing in place or pressure by thumb or finger can stop small bleeds.
- If bleeding is not controlled by initial dressing, apply a second pad and bandage over first.

> Not to remove the pad /dressing.

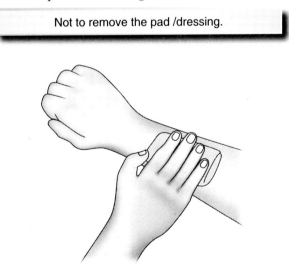

Fig. 3.23: Never remove pad/dressing

Remove the clothing from around the upper part of limb.

In case of uncontrolled bleeding (Fig. 3.24).

If direct pressure doesn't stop bleeding, consider applying a *constrictive bandage*.

> Constrictive bandages are a *last resort* and should only be attempted once all other avenues of stopping the blood loss have been exhausted.

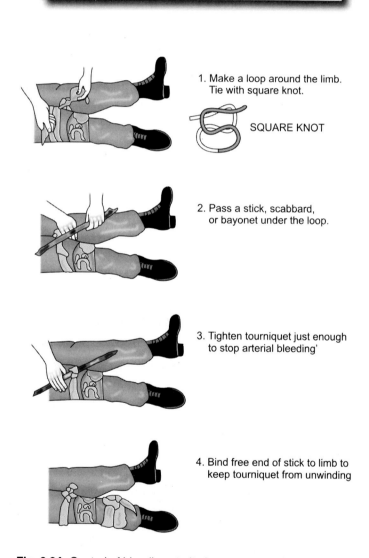

1. Make a loop around the limb. Tie with square knot.

   SQUARE KNOT

2. Pass a stick, scabbard, or bayonet under the loop.

3. Tighten tourniquet just enough to stop arterial bleeding'

4. Bind free end of stick to limb to keep tourniquet from unwinding

Fig. 3.24: Control of bleeding at site by custom-made tourniquet

- Thorough wash and dressing.
- *Splints,* if bleeding is from open fracture sites in extremities in form of whatever available stick, wood.
- *Tourniquets:* Is a temporary last resort on site to control bleeding with stick, bayonet or scabbard and make a loop around the limb and tie with square knot.

Internal / *invisible* loss can be controlled by

- Splints
- Rest to the part.

Disability (Neurological Evaluation)

As a first aid provider, you should always take head injury seriously

Check for

- Patients response
- Bleeding scalp
- Altered consciousness
- History of the incident
- Mechanism of injury.

Decide whether injury is

- *Life threatening*—Subarachnoid hemorrhage, internal damage to brain.
- *Life disabilitating*—Fracture skull, scalp injury.

Concussion is closed head injury, is often underestimated and injured succumb several hours after incident.

How to manage head injury at site?

Medical treatment begins from site itself.

Tricks

Immobilize—To prevent further damage to spine and nervous system

Apply pressure—It bleeds heavily in scalp, so apply pressure with thumb or hand for small wound and with bandage or instrument for large wound.

> No head injury is simple, so never never take head injury lightly.

If patient with head injury walks, talks ..... Don't think everything is fine.

It could be lull before a storm.

Or if patient is violent, it could be recovery or just brain irritability.

Applying bandage over head (Fig. 3.25)

It is just like tying to hold ball with string, dressing may slip or come out, so it is an art.

Apply knot in front or back, or with safety pin.

Shift to hospital.

Exposure

"If you don't look you won't see!"

Expose the patient to rule out associated injuries.

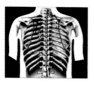

Secondary Survey

As CPR is in progress have view at other injuries which hampers prognosis of resuscitation.

Chest Injury

Have an ultra-quick look at chest for sucking wound, bruise over chest, impelled object, pain or difficulty in

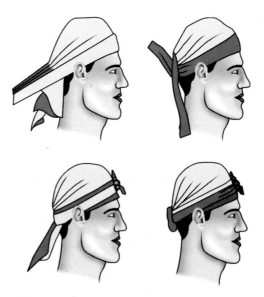

Fig. 3.25: Applying bandage for head injury

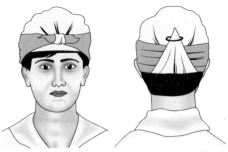

Fig. 3.26: Front and back view of bandage

breathing on affected site, brief about mechanism of injury, tenderness, crepitus on chest wall, deformity.

Reach the provisional diagnosis and treat it accordingly with the following:

First Aid Tricks

- Keep patient in **comfortable position** that is, **semi-reclining or semi-Fowler position** to avoid fight against gravity .
- Do not remove embedded object (Figs 3.27 and 3.28).
- Cover the sucking wound with occlusive dressing, field dressing, pressure dressing made airtight with clean plastic sheet or petroleum jelly, credit cards or available thing. Small opening known as flutter valve may be left open, so air can escape while lung reinflate (Fig. 3.29).
- Firm bandage over flail chest.
- For fractures immobilization in form of sling, braces, belts.
- Transfer in comfortable sitting position, oxygenation
- Reassurance.

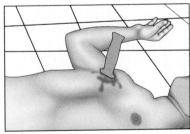
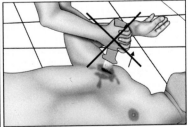

Fig. 3.27: Not to remove embedded object

Fig. 3.28: Not to remove embedded object

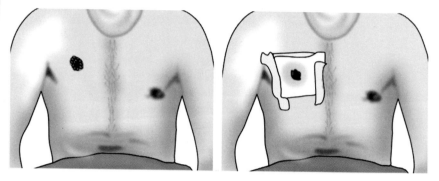

Fig. 3.29: Occlusive dressing

Abdominal Injury

View for abdominal wound, pain, vomiting, nausea, guarding, rigidity, evisceration, palpable fracture and associated injury.

What's up in tips and tricks in first aid?

- **Position**—Place injured person on their side in comfortable position since abdominal injury prompt vomiting, by placing person on one side it will allow them to expel the vomit with less likelihood of choking.
- Not to eat/drink.
- Don't remove penetrating object on site as it will further damage the damaged organ (Fig. 3.30).
- Instead stabilize object and put bulky dressing around the object as it may prevent an object from moving or being driven in deeper (Doughnut's dressing).

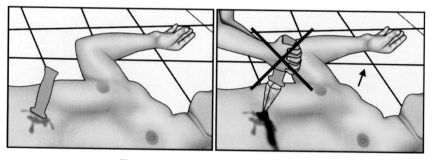

Fig. 3.30: Not to remove embedded object

- Dressing will help to control bleeding, prevent infection and contamination as well as absorb blood and drainage of wound.
- Never remove blood soaked dressing, rather add a layer of new clean dressing material.
- In case, if abdominal wound has resulted in causing protruding organ, do not attempt to reinsert the organ into the victim's body, this action could possibly damage the intestine and introduce infection in body.
- Don't cover it tightly with dressing, not to use fluffy cotton or cotton balls, as it's a poor choice of dressing material, because they contain fibers that can get into the wound causing difficulty upon removal. Clean nonadherent, washed cloth or towel which is larger than wound itself would be acceptable material (Fig. 3.31).
- Use drinkable water and pour it on the dressing to keep organ from drying out until tertiary center reached

Deep penetrating foreign body should remain in situ until theater exploration.

Pelvic Injury

It is life-threatening injury, so quickly see for palpable fracture, hematuria, tenderness, unable to weight bear or walk.

Tip   Don't manipulate pelvic fracture as it will bleed as much as 2 to 3 liters of blood.

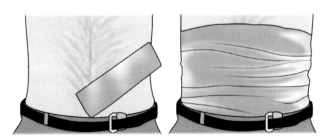

Fig. 3.31: Bulky or occlusive dressing

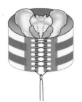

If suspected , use of *Pelvic binder* (wrapping a sheet around the pelvis and pulling this tight to close the open book fracture) can decrease blood loss.

Spine Injury

It is quite often missed, so most important is look for movements of all limbs and pinch, examine for back as mentioned with logroll method for bruise, tenderness, deformity.

Never neglect spinal injury particularly if there is head injury.

Cervical spine injury is the most common amongst it. Any further damage to spine can worsen neurological prognosis resulting in death or disability.

Tip   Immobilize cervical spine.

Fracture

How to diagnose fracture?

It is easily diagnosed with deformity, bleeding, wound, crepitus, edema.

How to manage fracture at site?

Initial fracture management can be given as mentioned below with help of mnemonic "PRICE".

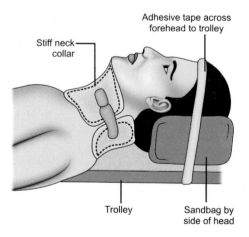

Fig. 3.32: Sandbag to support

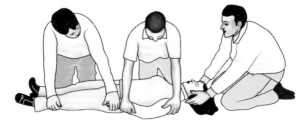

Fig. 3.33: Logroll method

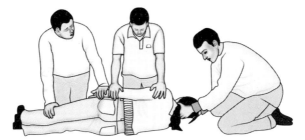

Fig. 3.34: Roll over position with cervical immobilization

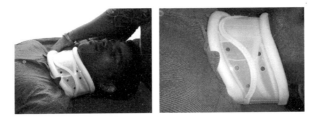

Fig. 3.35: Cervical collar

- **Prevention of fracture** damaging soft tissue.
- **Rest**—Helps to decrease bleeding/swelling and prevents injury to become worse.
- **Ice**—Causes vasoconstriction, resulting in decrease in blood flow, decrease in pain and swelling
- **Compression**—It limits swelling, maintains blood flow to injured part with help of crepe bandage.
- **Elevation**—Raising above heart, reduces the blood flow to injured part.

For ice application always use cloth/ handkerchief, never apply directly to skin, as it will further damage the tissue.

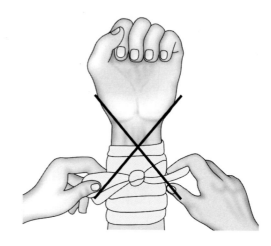

Fig. 3.36: Not to apply knot

Tip

Never massage the traumatized soft tissue.

Immobilization is the preferred way to manage fracture limbs, as it helps to:

- Reduce movement
- Reduce pain
- Reduce bleeding
- Reduce injury to surrounding structure like nerve, blood vessels, muscles.

Immobilization can be given with bandage and any available form like stick, cardboard, wooden or air splint.

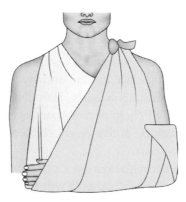

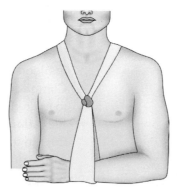

Fig. 3.37: Triangular sling   **Fig. 3.38:** Simple sling

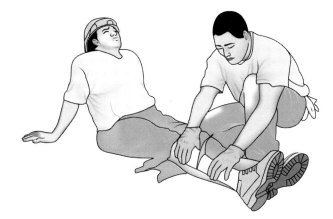

Fig. 3.39: Dressing being kept and bandage apply

Put dressing over exposed wound and do not apply tight bandage.

> Do not apply tight bandage, it will swell up limb.

Give sling and splint for upper extremity.

> Please, please check for distal circulation after splintage, as absent pulsation can lead to disastrous condition like amputation of limb.

If distal pulsation is absent, if you are experienced enough, gently and carefully try to align the bone with mild traction and splint before transfer.

> Do not try dislocated joint to relocate without guidance of expert, as it will further damage or fracture limb.

Do not bandage to fracture jaw—support jaw with hand and lean forward slightly or bandage it as shown below (Fig. 3.40).

How to know bandage is tight?

If,
- Pain, swelling
- Tingling, numbness in fingers / toes
- Absent distal pulsation
- Pale blue appearance below the bandage.

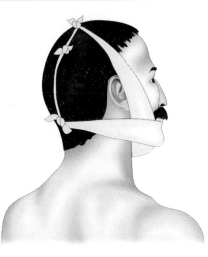

Fig. 3.40: Bandage for fractured jaw

How to treat tight bandage?

Immediate treatment is to release the bandage or make it loose. If circulation is fine, continue transport.

Crush Injury

- It occurs in situation like crushed by a car, earthquakes, falling masonry, trench cave, a mine shaft collapse.
- Prolonged pressure due to body weight in an unconscious patient.
- Injured appear alert and unduly distressed, however severe and irreversible damage may have been sustained and condition may deteriorate.
- The blood that is trapped and stationary by crushing object becomes toxic to heart, unless it is allowed to circulate again.

What to look for?

- Site—crushing forces across large muscle group—arms, thigh, back.
- Minimal pain, bruise.
- Sign of shock.

How to treat initially?

- Remove the crushing forces as early as possible.
- Monitor breathing and circulation.

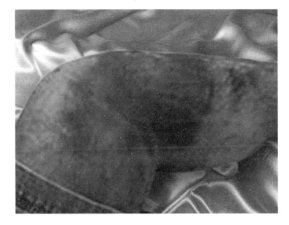

Fig. 3.41: Bruise over upper end tibia
(*For color version, see Plate 2*)

- Treat bleeding and fracture once crushing object is removed.
- Call ambulance.
- Prepare and continue CPR.
- Alert for renal failure—common.

> Do not apply tourniquet for first aid in management of crush injury.

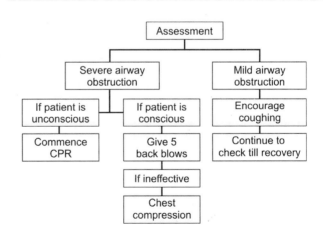

Fig. 3.42: Summary of trauma management at site

Preparation for Transport

Call Ambulance

- Give exact address in detail, i.e. street, nearest cross road, city/town, landmarks, it will help to arrive fast and easily.
- Caller name
- Phone number
- What happened or event occur, in short—car accident, fire, etc.
- Number of injured and level of consciousness, breathing, and circulation.
- Reassurance is of psychological value, and is important in first aid.
- If possible treating person should escort with crew members or should give detail information of what has been done and brief them about incidence, history, treatment given and status of patient.

CHAPTER 4

Management During Transport

- ➲ Transport of Trauma Patient
  - ○ How to Transport?
  - ○ Who can do It?
- ➲ Equipments and Monitoring
  - ○ What Facilities should be there in the Ambulance?
- ➲ Management and Survey
  - ○ Airway
  - ○ Breathing
    - • Intubation
    - • Tips and Tricks in Intubation
    - • Tips and Tricks in Difficult Intubation
  - ○ Circulation
    - • What is Automatic External Defibrillator (AED)?
    - • What Care is taken While Performing AED?
  - ○ Disability
  - ○ Exposure
  - ○ Management of Head Injury
  - ○ How to Manage Wound Care?
- ➲ Pitfalls in Transportation

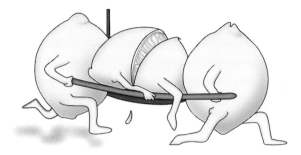

Fig. 4.1: Transport of ill patient

The transport of critically ill patient carries inherent risk. This risk can be minimized and outcome can be improved with careful planning and use of qualified personnel, selection and availability of equipments (Fig. 4.1).

No hiatus in monitoring and maintaining vital function of patient.

Transport of Trauma Patient

Multiple badly injured patient should reach the tertiary care in timely fashion to avoid a preventable death due to airway obstruction/ shock.

How to Transport?

Transport can be done in available form like airlift, road, or water.

Who Can Do It?

In early 20th century ambulance crew used to drove patient to nearest hospital, now emergency medical technician (EMT) has replaced it.

EMT—Emergency medical technicians are trained manpower like the anesthesia technician. They must have completed course of training and recertify every 2 to 4 years, they should be taught first aid and basic trauma life support skills in all age groups of trauma.

Their functions are as follow:
• They assess the scene, inform hospital about type of response required.
• EMT swiftly and safely extricate the patient with spinal precaution on backboard, this procedures

perform under physician supervision via radio or cellular contact.

- Do triage
- Patient assessment
- Help in transportation
- Perform basic skill mentioned below
  - Airway management
  - Hemorrhage control
  - Cardiopulmonary resuscitation
  - Artificial external defibrillator
  - Endotracheal intubation
  - Bag-valve-mask ventilation
  - Obtain IV access
  - Able to use portable monitors and ventilators
  - Treat shock
  - Stabilization of fractures.

Nurses should be well-trained to recognize emergency and skilled procedure like intubation, needle cricothyroidotomy and assist in same, maintain and introduce IV access, CV line, intraosseous line, and familiar with ventilator.

Ambulance

Ambulance driver.

What are the functions of ambulance driver?

- After receiving call, drives ambulance to the address given.
- Parks ambulance in a safe location
- If police are present, receives a briefing from them.
- Take over first responder.
- Take help of police or bystander.
- Assist EMT, it is good to have two team members, that is one—driver and two—EMT.
- Knowledge for basic trauma management.
- Familiar to the area for fast transport.

> Used logroll method for transport.

Ideal method for transport is four-person logroll method.

Following are four steps of logroll method (Fig. 4.2):
1. Immobilize the cervical spine.
2. Crew members kneel on one side of person and with hand placed on far side of injured.
3. On command examine the spine and slide the back board under the patient and roll patient on the board.
4. Centralize the patient and apply the belt.

Transport team should have knowledge of aerospace medicine, high altitude physiology, aircraft safety, airway communications.

On or off line physician 24 × 7 should be present to guide EMT.

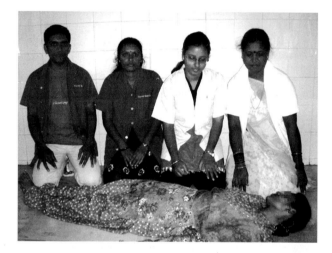

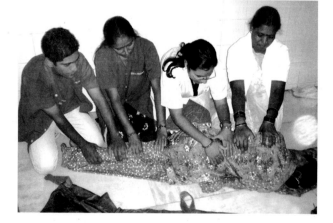

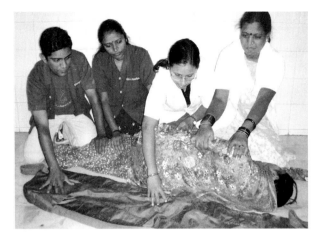

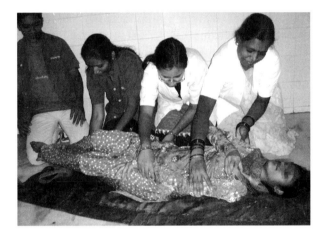

Fig. 4.2: Logroll method for transport
(*For color version, see Plates 2 and 3*)

Equipments and Monitoring

What Facilities should be there in Ambulance?

- Foldable stretcher for easy collection of injured.
- Oxygen trolley with equipments and back up facility.
- Necessary power converter, battery back up during transport for all equipments.
- Climate control ambulance.
- Monitoring devices—NIBP, pulse oximetry, ECG, ventilators, communicating devices—radio or satellite phones, defibrillators, PPE for EMT, extrication kit (Fig. 4.3).

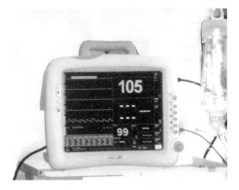

Fig. 4.3: Monitor (*For color version, see Plate 3*)

- NIBP (noninvasive blood pressure monitoring system) is particularly useful during transport as ambient noise may interfere by use of conventional sphygmomanometer.
- Userfriendly ventilator is used.

Management and Survey

Transport is best time to get some detail history and assessment of patient. The goal of initial assessment is to determine those injuries that threaten patient's life and if performed correctly it saves lives too.

Primary survey is known as ABCDE. Advanced trauma life support begins from transport itself (Fig. 4.4).

Airway

Injured patient may require advanced airway management during further transport. After assessing airway obstruction, consider following steps:
- Chin lift/jaw thrust
- Suctioning
- Guided airway/nasopharyngeal airway
- Intubation and reintubation itself must be prepared
- Laryngeal mask should be available, if intubation cannot take place
- Needle cricothrotomy by trained personnel may be useful in case of failed intubation.

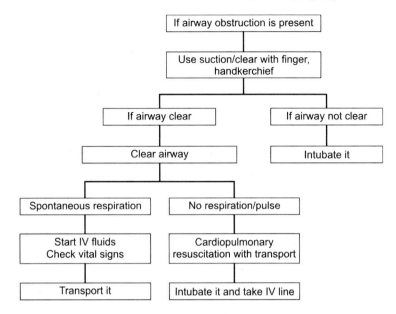

Fig. 4.4: Flow chart of ABC during transport

Breathing

If inadequate, look for
- Artificial ventilation
- Decompression and drainage of tension pneumothorax with either needle or chest tube thoracotomy by experts.
- Closure of open chest wound.
- Insert nasogastric tube, to prevent aspiration.
- Rate and method of oxygen administration.

Intubation

Position yourself.

Ensure everything is ready and patient is not breathing.

Keep this intubation kit / tray ready (Figs 4.5 and 4.6)
- Endotracheal tube of all size with guide wire
- Jelly, gloves
- Laryngoscope—check for battery, scope, blades of different size.
- Ambubag

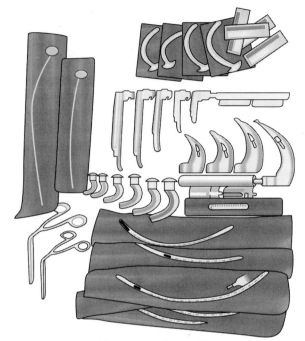

Fig. 4.5: Intubation kit

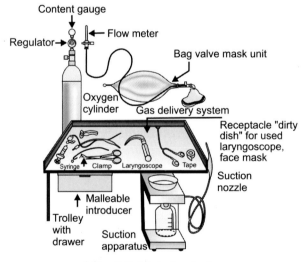

Fig. 4.6: Intubation trolley

- Facemask
- Airway
- Magill's forceps
- Plain syringe and tape for tube fixation
- Stethoscope.

Tips of Intubation

- Look for any nasal, coracoid fracture, denture, padiki, panmasala, chewing gum in mouth, if present, remove cause or do it with precaution.
- Check for respiration before intubation too.
- In obese patient it will be difficult to intubate as short neck will not allow to hyperextend further and because of obesity cricoid will not be seen.

Tricks of Intubation

- Flexion of neck can be achieved by putting doughnut or pillow under the head with extension of atlantoaxial joint.

- **Do not lose the sight of it while advancing laryngoscope (Fig. 4.8).**
- It is important to view vocal cord, if not viewed manipulate trachea with finger (Fig. 4.7).
- Use endotracheal tube of appropriate size in the right hand.

How to know tube is in?

- Fogging of ET tube on exhalation.
- Filling of reservoir bag on exhalation.
- Maintenance of arterial oxygenation.

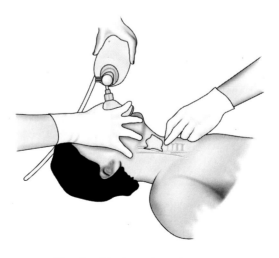

Fig. 4.7: Manipulation of trachea

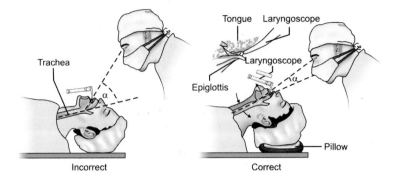

Fig. 4.8: Positioning on intubation

- On auscultation bilateral air entry.
- Chest X-ray.
- If the tube is not in the chest, tube is in the abdomen.

Tip

- Take care not to injure cricoid cartilage or trachea on repeated intubation as it will bleed and blood trickles in bronchi, further worsening situation.
- Tracheal intubation should be performed in no more than 30 seconds.
- If you are unable to intubate, continue ventilation of patient via mask.

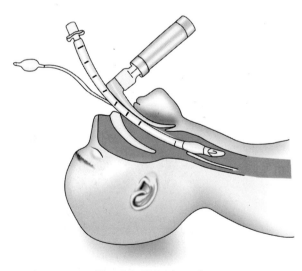

Fig. 4.9: Tube insertion

Remember patients die from lack of oxygen, not lack of an endotracheal tube.

If oral intubation not possible go for nasal or tracheostomy.

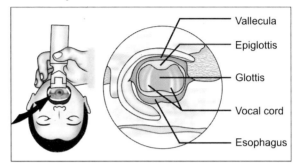

Fig. 4.10: Anatomical position

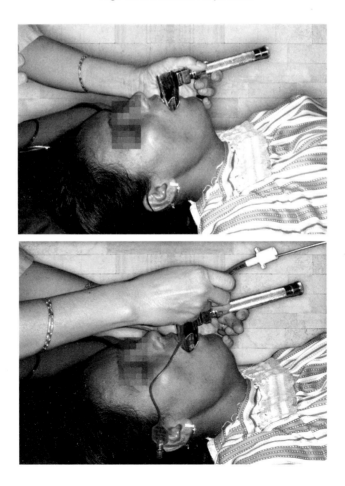

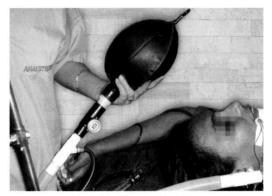

Fig. 4.11: Steps of intubation
(*For color version, see Plate 4*)

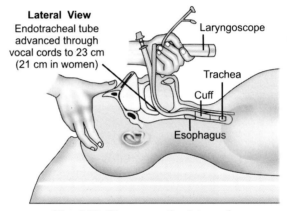

Fig. 4.12: Diagrammatic picture of scope,
position of tube and its level

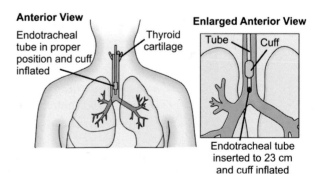

Fig. 4.13: Level of endotracheal tube

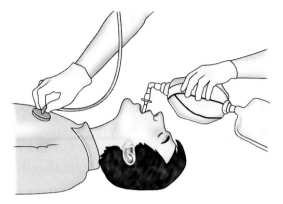

Fig. 4.14: Auscultate for bilateral air entry

Tips and tricks in difficult intubation

- In obese or long neck patient align ear with sternal notch in the horizontal plane. Use stylette and shape it straight to the cuff and only angle the tip. More curvature obscure the view.
- If larynx sited more anteriorly than usual do not hyperextend the neck during intubation, instead place a sandbag under the shoulders.
- Trick—flex the head, releasing strap muscles, this will allow larynx to be displaced backward using cricoid pressure.
- Use rigid bronchoscope if all this measures fail, call ear and neck surgeon to help out.

> With a difficult intubation never do anything you cannot get out of it.

Circulation

- Monitor vital signs
- Continue cardiorespiratory resuscitation support.
- Control bleeding as mentioned in next chapter.
- IV large bore cannula and crystalloid solution infusion.
- Restore blood volume, by blood volume replacement.
- Insert indwelling urinary catheter and monitor urine output.
- Monitor patient's cardiac rhythm and rate.

- Use of appropriate medicine like adrenaline, amiodarone, atropine, bicarbonate, calcium, potassium and magnesium under guidance of team captain.
- Maintain accurate records.

What is Automatic External Defibrillator?

It is device that corrects irregular or stopped heart beat by sending electrical shocks to the heart, to get back regular normal heart rhythm (Fig. 4.15).

What Care should be Taken while Performing AED?

- One shock followed by two minutes of CPR before going back to an AED.
- Never give two defibrillator together, give IV drugs, check for response and watch on monitor with ECG leads in situ.
- Check expiry dates of pads.
- Avoid touching patient while giving shock to avoid false reading.

Disability

Rapid neurological assessment, as there is no time to do the Glasgow coma scale, so use the following clear and quick system at this stage.

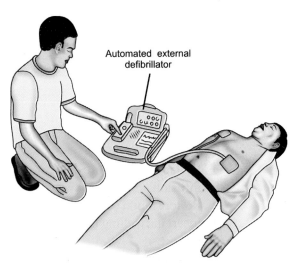

Automated external defibrillator

Fig. 4.15: Automatic external defibrillator

Check out

A – Awake

V – Verbal response

P – Painful response

U – Unresponsive.

Exposure of Patient

All trauma patient should be

- Completely exposed to identify all major injuries. Care must be taken not to cause further problems.
- Immobilize extremities, patients with unstable vital signs look out for the extremities fracture because of potential hemorrhage from long bones, which should be carefully splinted or traction may be given during transport, to prevent further damage and give greatest comfort during transport.

Management of Head Injury

- Immobilize the spine, head and neck. Monitor signs of intracranial pressure as mentioned in next chapter.

How to Manage Wound Care?

- Clean and dress, control bleeding with bandages.
- Best controlled by direct pressure and elevation above heart.
- Bandages that become soaked should not be removed, but rather reinforced with further bandage.
- Tourniquets should be used in life-threatening hemorrhage that cannot be controlled by direct pressure, elevation and bandaging.

Medication

Analgesia—Short acting parenteral agents like diclofenac, tramadol may be used.

Pitfalls in Transportation

- Distance
- Noise
- Vibration
- Lightening
- Altitude
- Weather sometimes interfere in treatment during transport.

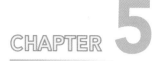

CHAPTER 5

Management at Hospitals/Tertiary Centers

Once patient is brought to hospital by ambulance crew or person, hospital staff take over and rapidly follow ABC's or continue CPR in hospital.

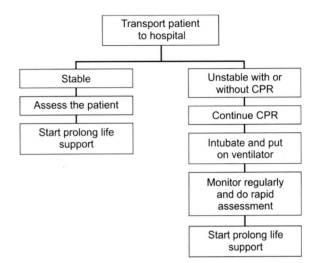

Fig. 5.1: Flow chart of management in hospital

Advance Trauma Life Support (ATLS)

What is ATLS?

The initial evaluation including **primary survey, resuscitation, secondary survey** and definite treatment or transfer of injured to tertiary care is heart of ATLS system, which is designed to identify life-threatening injuries and to initiate stabilizing treatment in a rapidly efficient manner.

What is their Goals?

To teach a simplified and standardized approach for trauma patient.

The basic goal of ATLS includes
- Concise method of assessment
- Interpretation of findings
- Initiate appropriate management based on priorities

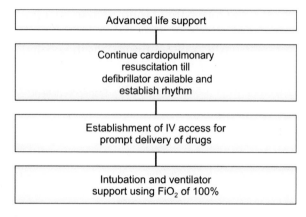

Advanced life support
Continue cardiopulmonary resuscitation till defibrillator available and establish rhythm
Establishment of IV access for prompt delivery of drugs
Intubation and ventilator support using FiO_2 of 100%

Fig. 5.2: Flow chart of ATLS

Primary Survey and Resuscitation

It is initial and key part of the assessment of patients presenting trauma is called the primary survey. It helps to identify life-threatening injuries and simultaneously resuscitation is begun.

A – Airway
B – Breathing
C – Circulation
D – Disability (Neurological Evaluation)
E – Exposure

Airway and Breathing

*"When you breathe you inspire
when you do not breathe, you expire".*

- Once the airway is established as mentioned previously.
- Give oxygenation by nasal prongs or by bag-valve-mask or by ventimask.
- If SpO_2 is not stabilized think of other obstruction like secretion, simple control of secretion by suctioning, endotracheal intubation or placement of surgical airway (cricothyroidotomy, tracheostomy) give 100% oxygen by same and monitor SpO_2 regularly.
- Cricothyroidotomy is emergency procedure, when intubation is unsuccessful and tracheostomy is not an option.

- Tracheostomy—A surgical procedure, for person, who requires long-term respiratory support.
- If still it is not stabilizing, put patient on mechanical ventilator give FiO_2 100%.

Once patient is able to ventilate by any of the above methods and breathing is secured immediately, look for circulation.

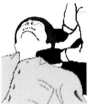

Circulation

- Oxygenated blood is important in circulation of human body.
- Irreversible brain injury or death can occur in few minutes of onset of cardiac standstill, so immediate treatment is mandatory.
- Take detail of vital. If patient is pulseless/ BP less/ shows signs of shock and if not responding to or minimal to basic life support then immediately give defibrillator.
- Defibrillator is a device used to deliver therapeutic dose of electrical energy to the affected heart. It depolarizes a critical mass of the heart muscle and allows normal sinus rhythm to reestablish by body.
- Defibrillators are started with 200 joules up to 360 joules can be given.

Tip

> Between each defibrillator give IV drugs like adrenaline and/or lidocaine and/or amiodarone to restore sinus rhythm.

Disability (Neurological Evaluation)

- This is done at the end of primary survey to determine the basic neurological assessment by using mnemonic **AVPU.**
  - Alert
  - Verbal command
  - Painful stimuli or
  - Unresponsive

This establishes the patient's level of conciousness, spinal cord injury level.

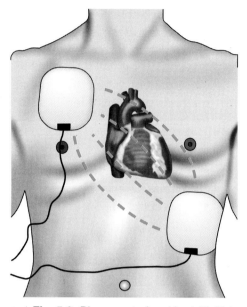

Fig. 5.3: Placement of pad in defibrillator

- An altered level of consciousness indicates the need for immediate reevaluation of patient's oxygenation, ventilation and perfusion status.

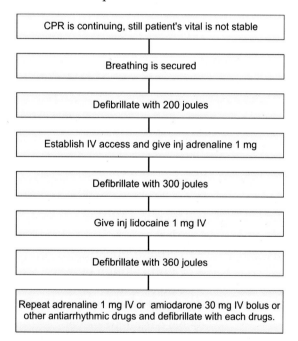

Fig. 5.4: Management using defibrillator

Exposure

You can't treat what you don't find!

This is the final step of primary survey.

Patient should be undressed, all garments, jewellary should be cut and removed.

Prevent hypothermia by prophylactic administration of warm IV fluids, blankets, heat lamps.

Maintain privacy of patient.

> Hypothermia can lead to abnormal blood clotting.

Dr Sejal's Principle of Prolong Life Support

Now once injured is stabilized, management of prolong life support begins.

Prolong life support includes following principles, with continuing resuscitative phase, secondary survey and rehabilitation.

Principle

a. To find cause of instability of organ or system injured.
b. To monitor and treat the injured system or organ.
c. To reverse the complication arising from CPR on site or during transport.
d. To start early rehabilitation.

What Makes Injured Still in Resuscitative Phase?

Is it,
- Shock?
- Ongoing bleeding from site of injury or organ?
- Damage to particular organ?

Shock

Marshall Hall in 1825 gave idea about maintaining circulatory blood volume and its effects on loss of blood.

It is a life-threatening condition.

It is a top priority, second to the ABC.

What is Shock?

Shock is defined as inadequate organ perfusion and tissue oxygenation.

In trauma patient, it is most often due to hemorrhage and hypovolemia.

Acute in onset, it is resulting from critical fall in capillary perfusion which reduces tissue oxygen delivery below its minimum nutrition needs and is incompatible with life if persists long.

How to know shock?

- Check peripheral pulses, capillary refill, and blood pressure.

  Tip-radial pulsation used or if not palpable-femoral, brachial, carotid should be checked. Reduction in systolic blood pressure below 90 mm of Hg.
- Noninvasive blood pressure monitoring system should be used particularly in children.
- Thirst, loss of blood, body fluids.
- Perspiration.
- Reduction of urine output below 20 ml/hour.

Signs	Healthy/normal	Shock
Skin condition	Pink, warm, dry	Pale, cold, wet
Conscious	Alert, aware of environment	Altered, confused, aggressive.
Pulse	Adult 60–100/min	Rapid above upper limit.
	Child 90–130/min	
	Infants 120–140/min	
Respiration	Adult 12–20/min	Rapid above upper limit.

If shock not timely managed or treated to neglectfulness complacency as reversible shock may develop into irreversible shock.

What can lead to shock in trauma management?

- Loss of blood
  - External—loss is from open fracture, stab abdomen, chest or bleeding head
  - Internal—from blunt abdomen, chest, head, pelvic, spine injury, closed fracture
  - Immediate/delay bleeding

- Loss of body fluids
- Spinal injury
- Crush injury – following land sliding, earthquakes, etc.

Remember

> - Large volumes of blood may be hidden in the abdominal and pleural cavity.
> - Femoral fracture loses up to 2 liters of blood.
> - Pelvic fracture often loses in excess of 2 liters of blood.

So, amount of blood loss after trauma is often poorly assessed and in blunt trauma is usually under estimated, resulting in **hemorrhagic shock.**

Sometimes in condition like penetrating wound to the heart, myocardial infarction, contusion, tamponade and tension pneumo-thorax, there is inadequate function of heart to pump result in **Cardiogenic shock.**

Due to the loss of sympathetic tone, usually resulting from spinal cord injury.

The classical presentation is hypotension without reflex tachycardia or skin vasoconstriction and **neurogenic shock** develops.

Rarely in the early phase but common during late phase of trauma (when multiorgan dysfunction occurs) **Septic shock** is seen.

> Hypovolemia is a life-threatening emergency and must be recognized and treated aggressively.

Bleeding

It is one of the culprits to develop disturbance in circulation and is explained in previous chapter.

Management of Shock and Bleeding

Ask yourself,
- Does injury appear serious?
- If I don't respond, injured likely to become worse?
- Death is possibility?

If answer to any of these is *'yes'*, then you should treat shock.

Goal

How to stop bleeding and restore oxygen delivery to the tissues?

a. *External visible* loss can be controlled by

Apply **RED,** as mentioned, if not relieved then theater exploration with

- *Instruments*—if there is profuse external bleeding identify the bleeder or major vessels and tie up with artery or nonabsorbable suture material, clamps.
- *Tourniquets* as a temporary last resort, if all measures fail to control bleeding.

This is an emergency management and not a definitive management to prevent acute blood loss.

It should be applied properly with great care and time, proper pressure, and place to prevent further loss to other vital organs/tissue and limbs.

Pressure — upper limb – systolic BP + 50 mm Hg
—lower limb—twice systolic blood pressure

Time — upper limb one hour and twenty min. Lower limb one hour and forty min.

Place — it should not be over joint, it should be at a place with good musculature like thigh and arms.

Tips in Tourniquet

- Check working of tourniquet and tubing, equipments properly.
- Check for all cuffs including pediatric.
- Wall clock.
- Proper padding to prevent skin ischemia.

Complications like skin necrosis, gangrene to part, nerves, muscle, vessels are seen.

Tip

Do not attempt to control minor bleeding or minor injuries during initial assessment. Only bleeding, that is life-threatening is to be controlled.

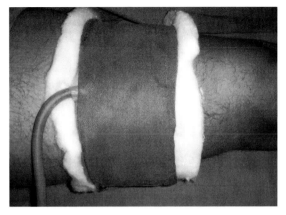

Fig. 5.5: Positioning and padding of tourniquet

b. *Internal/invisible* loss can be controlled by
  • Splints and braces
  • Immobilization/traction
  • Rest to the part
  • Operation/instrument/procedures.
c. Other
  • Reassurance – allaying anxiety – leads to sympathetic over activity, vaso-constriction, tachycardia, tachypnea, nausea and vomiting, shallow breathing.
  • Do not overheat, maintain body temperature.
  • Cessation of ongoing insult by
    Obtaining adequate vascular access and obtain samples using at least two large bore cannulas (14–16 G).
  • Initial treatment of hypovolemia is by rapid infusion of a ringer lactate solution via two large bore peripheral IV catheters or central venous line.

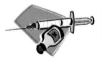

IV line preferably in upper limb or central venous line.

Take two IV line, 1st IV line draw blood for investigation and for no delay start IV fluids in 2nd IV line.

Tips

IV fluid should be given with caution particularly in geriatric, pediatric and cardiac compromised person, as it will cause cardiac overload and further worsen situation.

- Treatment of hypoglycemia, acidosis
- *Treatment of cause.*

> Avoid solution containing glucose.

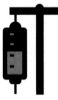

When should blood transfusion be considered?

- If uncontrollable bleeding, unrecoverable shock.
- If when fluid like crystalloid and colloid infusion fails to stabilize hemodynamically.
- If hemoglobin is less than 7 gm/dl and patient is still bleeding. If type specific or cross matched blood is not available, **use group O negative packed red blood cell.**

> Any of the fluid should be warm before administering.

Increase organ flow by the drugs which increase cardiac contractility producing vasodilatation like digitalis, glucagon, dopamine.

Treat cardiac tamponade by pericardio-centesis followed by surgical exploration and control of bleeding.

Other Procedures Like

- *ECG, ventilatory* lead monitoring, pulse oximetry monitoring should take place simultaneously.
- *Nasogastric tube* to decompress the stomach and lessen the likelihood of aspiration of gastric contents.
- Insert a *Foley's catheter* to measure the response to fluid resuscitation.

Tips

> Urinary catheterization should be done with precaution in case of urethral injury or pelvic injury.

Pathological Tests

- Get done base line (complete blood count, urinalysis, serum electrolytes, clotting studies, blood group type and cross match, HIV and HbsAg) "trauma package"—as a practical purpose, so that you don't forget something important.

To Summarize Resuscitative Phase

- During the primary survey, when making diagnosis and performing interventions, until the patient condition is stabilized, diagnostic workup, resuscitative procedure and surgeries is completed. The ongoing efforts involve monitoring patient vital signs, protecting airway with assisted ventilation and oxygenation and resuscitation with IV fluids and blood products, antibiotics.
- Patient with polytrauma requires large amount of crystalloids over the first 24 hours of injury to sustain intravascular volume, tissue and vital organ perfusion and urine output.
- Administer blood volume in case of unresponsive hypovolemia to crystalloid bolus.
- Blood lactate and blood gases level may be helpful in severely injured to get feedback for oxygenation, ventilation and tissue perfusion.

In short, management of hospital can be remembered by following H's (Dr Sejal's criteria):

- Hypoxia
- Hypovolemia
- Hyperkalemia or hypokalemia (abnormal potassium in the blood) and associated abnormal calcium and magnesium levels.
- Hypothermia
- Hydrogen ions (acidosis)
- Hypoglycemia

a. **How to monitor and treat the injured system or organ**—as mentioned in next chapter.

b. **Which are complications arising from the resuscitative phase?**

   Complication may worsened the ongoing condition, which is tackled accordingly during this phase.

   It is common that you make mistake and complication arises from the same.

   So, look for the same while you are treating the emergencies.

At site

- *Faulty bandaging technique* – Improper bandaging results in bleeding, slipping during transfer, increase in pain if not snugly fitted.
- *Are you injuring* to nose, tooth, lips, face eyes and injury to cervical spine while checking for airway obstruction or minimally manipulation on removing helmet?
- *Are you disturbing distal neurovascular* status or Gangrene following tight bandaging or splinting in fracture in extremities?
- Is *bleeding uncontrollable* because of self-injury to trachea, mouth or bleeding wound, manipulation of fracture, dressing not done?
- *Oh no,* I remove the penetrating object which can cause further bleeding, injury to organ and evisceration of injured organ.
- *What are you doing?* Keeping the eviscerated organs back.
- *Are you running?* Hasty and fast CPR, results in injury to ribs, upper abdominal organ, lungs, further add the complication and prolong the resuscitative phase.
- *No attempt to reduce* fracture/dislocation by nonexpert person results in further fracture and injury to surrounding joint, nerves, vessels, muscle.
- *Sudden* cardiac arrest, pulmonary/fat embolism, later renal failure.
- *Infection* because of dirt and improper padding or dressing.
- *I forget to look for other injuries.*

c. **Rehabilitation is as mentioned in next chapter.**

CHAPTER 6

Management of Traumatized System at Hospital

- ➲ Head Injury
  - ○ Why Head Injury?
  - ○ Tips to Evaluate Head Injury
  - ○ How to Determine Severity of Head Injury?
  - ○ What are Investigation to be Done?
  - ○ How will You Know Increase in Intracranial Pressure?
  - ○ How to Manage Head Injury?
  - ○ Recent Advances in Head Injury
- ➲ Chest Injury
  - ○ Tips to Evaluate Chest Injury
  - ○ What to Investigate?
  - ○ How to Treat?
- ➲ Abdominal Injury
  - ○ Tips to Evaluate Abdomen Injury
  - ○ What to Investigate?
  - ○ How shall I Treat It?
- ➲ Pelvic Injury
  - ○ Why Life-threatening ?
  - ○ Mechanism of Injury
  - ○ How to Diagnose?
  - ○ What to Investigate?
  - ○ How to Manage?
- ➲ Spinal Injury
  - ○ Tip of How to Evaluate Spinal Injury?
  - ○ Management
    - • Can you Treat Spinal Cord Injury? How?
    - • What is the Aim?
    - • What are Goals of Conservative Management?
- ➲ Fractures
  - ○ Tips for How to Evaluate?
  - ○ Don't Crack the Treatment…. Just Fix it.
    - • Conservative
    - • Surgical
  - ○ Fracture in Elderly and in Children.

Secondary Survey

It begins after completing the primary survey, after starting resuscitation phase. At this time identify all injuries from head to toe.

Best time to take history of trauma patient is between initial stabilization and secondary examination get some information from EMT's, paramedics, relatives about accident scene, past surgical/medical history, last meal, allergies, mode of injury.

Review the patient vital signs and perform quick repeat primary survey to assess the patient response to the resuscitation effort and to identify any deterioration.

The one of dicta for physical examination *"finger or tubes in every orifice"*.

In case of polytrauma more than one system may be affected and should not be neglected.

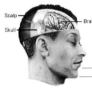

Head Injury

In any organization, head is the chief governing body, whether organization is man made or God made.

Like so, head is very important chief governing vital organ of our body.

Why Head Injury?

Injury to chief organ can lead to disturbance to other organs resulting in death of the body.

Brain is hard disc of our body, it stores memory, governs body, takes decision, guides body.

Importance of head injury came into existence during automobile era of trauma.

Age group—15 to 35 years

Sex—male >female

Tips to Evaluate Head Injury

Presentation depends and varies upon injury
- **Loss, altered level of consciousness**
- **Seizure**
- **CSF leaks ear, nose, throat is a conclusion of head injury**

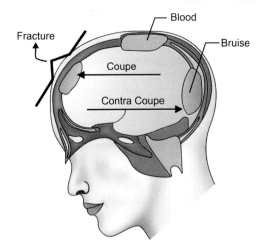

Fig. 6.1: Closed head injury

On Examination

- Rapid history, mode of injury, impact of injury.
- Eyes-pupils BERL (Bilateral equally reacting to light).
- Look for eye, ear, skull, nasal, facial bone (black eye), cervical spine, for fracture, dislocation, bleeding, injury.
- Neurological status by Glasgow coma scale in detail as mentioned below.
- Once scale taken, examination finished and provisional diagnosis achieved go for necessary investigation as mentioned below.

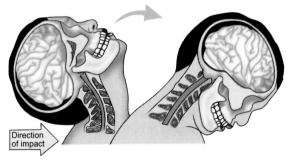

On sudden backward movement of skull in hyperextended cervical spine results in striking of brain in front

In Hyperflexed cervical spine head stops & brain impacts back on occiput

Fig. 6.2: Mode of injury

	1	2	3	4	5	6
Eyes	Does not open eyes	Open eyes in response to painful stimuli	Open eyes in response to voice	Open eyes spontaneously	N/A	N/A
Verbal	Makes no sounds	Incomprehensible sounds	Utters inappropriate words	Confused disoriented	Oriented, converses normally	N/A
Motor	Makes no movements	Extension to painful stimuli	Abnormal flexion to pain stimuli	Flexion/withdrawal to painful stimuli	Localizes painful stimuli	Obeys commands.

How to Determine Severity of Head Injury?

Glasgow Coma Scale

It is Universal system of identifying severity of traumatic brain injury, Glasgow coma scale comprises three tests— eye, verbal, motor command.

According to severity, grades and level of consciousness on a scale of 3 to 15 based on

Glasgow coma scale 13 or ≥ mild

9 to 12 moderate

≤ 8 severe

*Pediatric Glasgow coma scale a*s described in chapter of pediatric trauma.

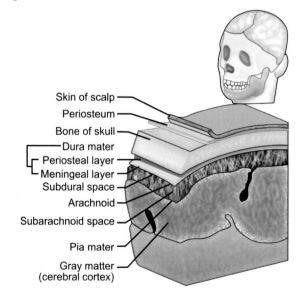

Skin of scalp
Periosteum
Bone of skull
Dura mater
Periosteal layer
Meningeal layer
Subdural space
Arachnoid
Subarachnoid space
Pia mater
Gray matter (cerebral cortex)

Fig. 6.3: Cross-section of skull and brain

Head injury can be of

- Extra-axial occurring within skull but outside brain tissue, includes (Figs 6.4 and 6.5)
  - Epidural hematoma
  - Subarachnoid hemorrhage
  - Subdural hematoma
  - Intracranial hemorrhage
- Intra-axial occurring within brain tissue
  It can be,
  - Focal—hemiparesis, aphasia, etc.
  - Diffuse—concussion, axonal injury.

What are Investigations to be Done?

Special investigation should be done
- Once patient is stable
- Information desired from previous investigation is insufficient
- To determine next step of therapy.

X-ray—not much useful tool.

CT scan (Recommended)—quick, accurate, widely available.

Follow-up CT may be performed for prognosis of injury.

MRI—help to know long-term status in axonal, diffuse injury, but not helpful in emergency.

Angiography useful in penetrating injury ophthalmic, ENT, Orthopedic examination.

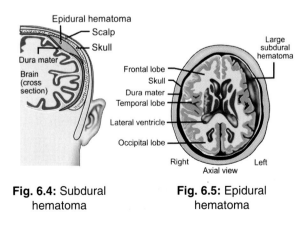

Fig. 6.4: Subdural hematoma

Fig. 6.5: Epidural hematoma

How will you know Increased Intracranial Pressure?

Traumatic brain injury occurs more frequently because of alteration in cerebral blood flow and pressure within skull.

> • Decreased level of consciousness.
> • Paralysis or weakness on one side of body.
> • Blown pupil—fail to constrict with light or slow to light.
> • Slow heart rate and high blood pressure.
> • Respiratory depression.

How to Manage Head Injury?

Head Injury is Enigma

• Unfortunately, once the brain has been damaged by trauma, there is **no quick fix.**
• Good looking, calm head injury can be **grevious injury.**
• Small clot may bleed up to 72 hours post- injury and causes disaster to patient, so explain seriousness of head injury to them, take proper consent.
• If left untreated many patients develop complication, which leads to death or permanent disability.

> Do not allow concussed injured head to "PLAY ON".

Tips in Prevention of Head Injury

• Seat belts, child seats, airbag are important to prevent head injury in road traffic accident.
• Installing grab bars in bathroom or handrails on staircase for geriatrics.
• Safety helmets for machine industry, mine workers, laborers, sports person.
• Fall can be avoided installing window guard, safety gates on top and bottom of stairs for young children.
• Soft ground surface like mulch or sand for children.
• Keep guns unloaded and lock.
• Changes into public policy and safety laws including speed limit, road engineering practice, etc.
• Improvement in equipments, headgear particularly in soccer—for heading.

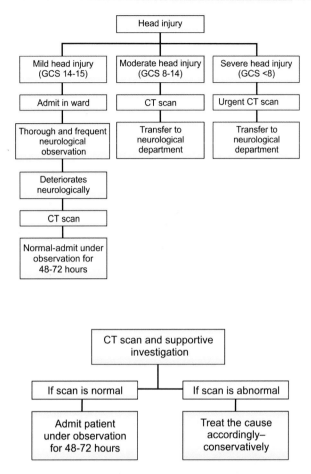

Fig. 6.6: Management of head injury

Tips of How to Treat in Hospital?

- After bleeding is secured and patient is conscious and cooperative rapid physical examination.
- In head injury, explain prognosis to patient's relatives.
- Sedation, paralytics, CSF diversion, diuretics to reduce excess fluids in the system, it can cause hypovolemia.
- Hyperventilation causes decrease in CO_2 levels and causes constriction of blood vessels results in decrease blood flow to brain and decrease intracranial pressure.
- Epsolinise patient if convulsion present

- Injection mannitol—to reduce brain edema controversial?
- Injection antiemetic, antacids
- Hypothermia–Temperature should be carefully regulated as increase in temperature increases brain metabolic needs.
- Blood pressure can be kept at artificially high level under controlled condition by infusion of norepinephrine or similar drug, it helps to maintain cerebral perfusion.
- Surgically—Decompression, craniotomy (Figs 6.7A to D).

What Important Discharging Tip You will Give to Relatives?

- Patient's relatives should be well-informed about convulsion, vomiting, bleeding, if present contact immediately to hospital.
- Keep patient under regular follow up for 6 to 12 weeks minimum.
- The caretakers of those patients with wild trauma when discharged from the hospital are frequently advised to **ROUSE** the patient several times during first 12 to 24 hours to assess worsening symptoms.

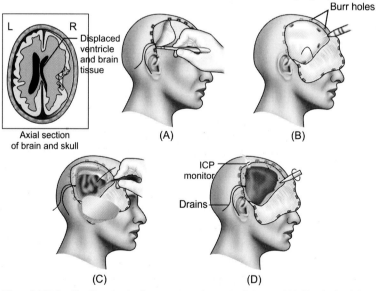

Figs 6.7A to D: Surgical- decompression craniotomy (A) Scalp incision (B) Multiple Burr holes (C) Subdural hemorrhage (D) Scalp flap secured in position

In addition to use of modern intensive care method, advances are due to monitoring of intracranial pressure directly, steroid therapy in very high doses (still controversial) and early activation in the subacute stage after injury.

Prevention of rise in intracranial pressure using monitoring allows appropriate intervention for intracranial head injuries and for preservation of the cerebral perfusion pressure.

The Most Common Errors in Head Injury Evaluation and Resuscitation are:

- Failure to perform ABC and prioritize management.
- Failure to look beyond the obvious head injury.
- Failure to assess the base line neurological examination.
- Failure to reevaluate a patient, who deteriorates.

> Never assume alcohol is the cause of drowsiness in a confused patient.

Some Fascinating Facts of Head Injury

Patient, who sustain head injury resulting to unconsciousness for an hour to few more hour have twice risk of developing Alzheimer disease later in life.

Chest Injury

Serious injury, it was first described in around 1600 BC in ancient Egyptian, Edwin Smith Papyrus.

Injury to chest in this automobile era following driving motor car, impact of steering in chest, leads to flail chest and death.

Tips to Evaluate

Apart from chest symptoms and signs, look for
- Pain on movement of chest during breathing/ coughing/stress.
- Crackling sound/feeling.

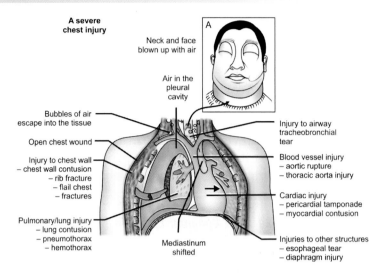

Fig. 6.8: Organ affecting chest injury

- Sucking chest wound-sound of air flowing through wound.
- Tachypnea, tachycardia.
- Tenderness at site on injury.

Tips on Examination

Inspection—if injured is breathing normally.
- Ask him to take deep breath, this attempt will soon be stopped by sharp pain, *fracture of ribs is confirmed*.
- Mediastinal shift can be known by feeling suprasternal notch, to find out if trachea is displaced.
- If intercostals distended on one side compared to other *(tension pneumothorax)*. unequal chest rise is seen.
- Whether air is going in and out and breathing is distressed or patient is still hungry for air (more respiratory effort) or he is cyanosed in presence of an adequate airway *(in case of damaged lung, flail chest, pneumothorax)*.
- *Anemic* patients do not become cyanosed and may die of anoxia without showing it. There must be 5 gm/dl of hemoglobin in circulation to observe cyanosis.
- Look for distended jugular veins *(anything which impedes venous return to heart like tension pneumothorax, mediastinal shift, cardiac tamponade)*.

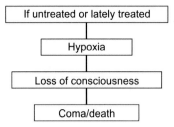

Fig. 6.9: Lately/untreated chest injury

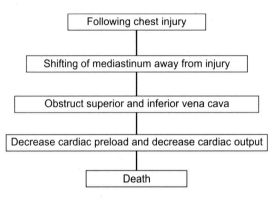

Fig. 6.10: Consequences following chest injury

Palpation—tenderness, crepitus—fractured ribs, crackling feeling of subcutaneous tissue suggesting of surgical emphysema.

Percussion should be done cautiously to prevent further damage, hyperesonance percussion note of chest wall on affected side.

Auscultate clicking sound for fractured ribs, coarse crepitation for surgical emphysema, reduced or absent breath sound on one side indicating fluid or air in pleural cavity, high pitched breath sounds suggestion of tension pneumothorax.

Recommended Investigations are

X-ray Chest

- Look out for multiple rib, clavicle fracture. Rib fracture at angle sometimes cannot be seen in AP X-rays, for this oblique view of right or left chest is taken.

- Shows large, globular swelling of heart.
- Look for old pathology, which can worsen the situation, particularly in geriatric patient.
- Collapsed lung, ventilated lung, hyper-ventilated lung, hazzy lung—effusion, hemo- pneumothorax.
- Diaphragm—air below diaphragm indicates perforation in GIT or pathological diaphragm.
- Look for CP angle—utmost important in case of early hemothorax.
- Quick look over surrounding joint like shoulder, acromioclavicular, clavicle.
- Shifting of mediastinum or aorta seen in pneumothorax.

HRCT scan (high resonance CT scan)

For evaluation lung pathology, thin sections with high spatial frequency reconstructions are used both in inspiration and expiration. This special technique is called HRCT.

- It is still evolving in chest injury.
- It confirms all radiological findings.
- Useful in aortic injuries, occasionally pneumome-diastinum, hemopericardium.
- CT pulmonary angiography (CTPA) is particularly useful in pulmonary embolism.

ECG – to rule out cardiac injury and overload.

Bronchoscopy

- To view airway abnormalities
- To clear secretions, blood or foreign objects lodged in the airway.
- To evaluate bleeding in the lung (collapse).
- To assist intubation in cases of difficult airway with flexible bronchoscope.

How to Treat?

Prevention Tips

- Body arm or made of rigid plates or other heavy material protects from projectiles generated in explosions.
- Chest garments—specially designed for military personnel, who are at high risk of blast injuries, to

prevent shock wave being propagated stress to chest wall or lung.

"Speed thrills, but it drills life."

So, use seat belts and airbags to prevent chest injury in this automobile era.

At Hospital

- After details of history, vitals and impact of trauma.
- Diagnose it with help of investigation, specialist.
- Position—Make patient to sit in semi-reclining position (Fig. 6.11).

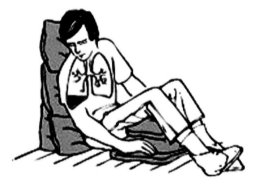

Fig. 6.11: Make patient sit in semi-reclining position

- Oxygenation and close monitoring needed with intervene care needed.
- If breathing is further impaired—mechanical ventilation required.
- Fluid replacement—take care for fluid overload—it may result in pulmonary edema.
- Lung contusion and chest wall contusion, which is commonly seen during blast injury.
  - Heals spontaneously with supportive care.
  - Closed monitoring and observation.
  - Oxygenation
  - IV fluids.
  - Antibiotics.
- Pericardial tamponade (fluid accumulate in pericardium), commonly following stab injury.

See it, feel it, diagnose it, and act it.

- Immediate IV line, if possible CVP (femoral or subclavian).

- IV fluids.
- Blood transfusion and replacements.
- Immediate shifting and preparation of operation theater for Thoracotomy (release of clotting in pericardium).
- Pneumothorax, hemothorax, release of intrathoracic pressure urgently by draining air, fluid by
    - needle thoracocentesis or tube thoracostomy (Figs 6.13A to C).

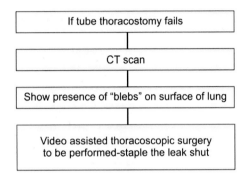

Fig. 6.12: Treatment to decrease intrathoracic pressure

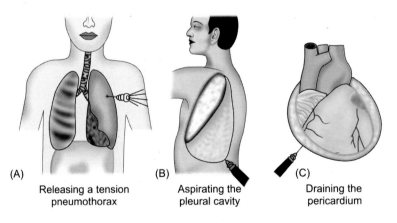

(A)	(B)	(C)
Releasing a tension pneumothorax	Aspirating the pleural cavity	Draining the pericardium

Figs 6.13A to C: Urgent method for chest decompression

Some Urgent Methods for Chest Injuries

Don't allow untreated pneumothorax to transport by flight –absolute contraindication.

Tube Thoracostomy

Tips and tricks

- Seal the tubing properly so that air cannot go in.
- Follow up repeat X-ray chest to know status of lung.
- Use flutter valve, which will not allow fluid or air to escape in pleural cavity.
- Tube should not be occluded with clot and other fibrinous material it will build up air in pleural space.
- Milk it, strip it or replace it, if clot present.
- Use large bore tube, smaller tube increase risk of clogging.
- Sign of chest tube clogging is surgical emphysema.
- Traumatic rupture of aorta—difficult to detect and usually go unnoticed.
  Diagnosis by aortography
  Treatment
  - Surgery
  - Look for associated injury like spinal cord ischemia leading to paraplegia
  - Prognosis—75-90 percent death occurs since bleeding is so profuse before reaching to tertiary care center.

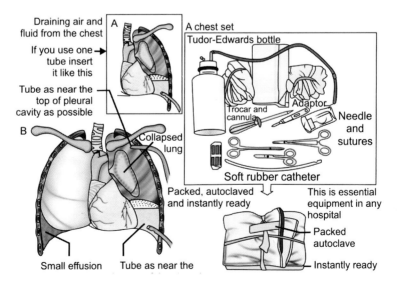

Fig. 6.14

- Fractures of chest
  Treatment for fracture of chest like ribs, clavicle, sternum and scapula (rare) (Fig. 6.15).

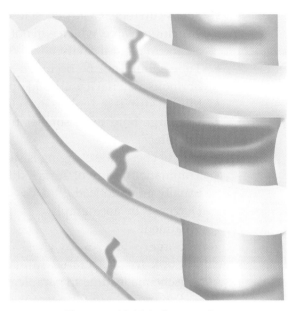

Fig. 6.15: Multiple fracture ribs

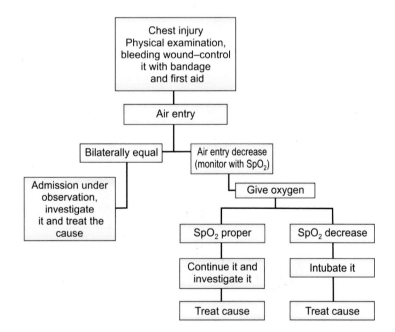

Fig. 6.16: Management of chest injury

– Immobilization in form of rest, oxygenation, different type of strapping, braces, slings.
– Surgery rarely required.

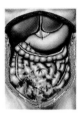

Abdominal Injury

- Blunt abdomen injury is a common cause of trauma following fall from height/accident.
- Spleen is most commonly involved in blunt abdomen.
- The liver is the commonest organ injured in penetrating trauma.
- Patient may come to you walking with abdominal pain or associated with multiple fractures or other injuries, **Don't neglect it.**

> The abdomen should neither be ignored nor the sole focus on.

It can be blunt or penetrating injury.
Causes:
- Road traffic accident
- Gunshot
- Stab/penetrating injury
- Child abuse

Tips to Evaluate

It is usually associated with other injury, penetrating injury is commonly seen.

Take in detail of history, particularly obstetric in female.
- Abdominal pain over injured site or organ.
- Tenderness, guarding, rigidity over the injured organ or whole abdomen.
- Abdominal distension usually after few hour.
- Bleeding P/R or P/V to rule out injury to bladder, urethra, uterus associated with hematuria.
- Decrease bowel sound.
- Evisceration (protruding of internal organ out of wound).

Beware

Abdominal injury is life-threatening in following conditions:

- Retroperitoneal space because of profuse blood loss (Fig. 6.17).
- Infection is common in late stage.
- Liver, spleen, kidney—bleed profusely following cut/torn.

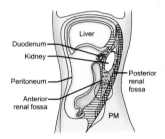

Fig. 6.17: Retroperitoneal space

Never

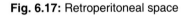

Neglect left lower rib fracture for splenic injury unless and until proven.

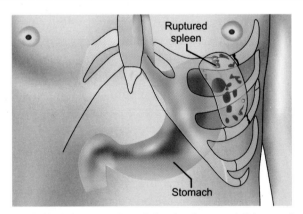

Fig. 6.18: Injury to spleen following fracture left lower ribs

Tips on Examination

Inspection—look for bruise, open wound, penetrating object, fullness or increase in size abdomen.

Palpation—guarding and rigidity in particularly quadrant or in general suggest injury/pathology to that particular organ.

Percussion- resonant note in fullness suggestive of free fluid in abdomen.

Auscultation—Listen for bowel sound.

No Examination of Abdomen is Completed without Per-rectal or Pervaginal Examination

In case of abdomen injury try to look and expose patient to see injury to genitalia, accordingly get involved gynecologist too.

"We had one case of unmarried teen girl, had an accident with blunt abdomen and unable to walk with bleeding genitalia, we settled patient, immediately examined , USG abdomen showed no abnormality, X-ray pelvis—fracture pubic rami, initially urine not passed, later in hour, she passed urine, admission was done. But she was still bleeding and blood pressure was decreasing slowly.

Gynecologist was consulted, she looked at it, externally there was no wound, gynecologist adviced examinaton under anesthesia. Per vaginam showed huge vaginal tear extending up to cervix, which was repaired and patient settled.

Retrogradely we took history, it was accident of scooter with bicycle, and bicycle steering pierced in and caused tear in whole vagina and cervix".

What to Investigate?

Objective

- Main is to identify for intra-abdominal free fluid using diagnostic peritoneal lavage (DPL) or focused assessment with sonography for trauma **(FAST).**
- To identify patients, who need a laparotomy.

X-ray

- Gas under diaphragm in case of bowel perforation.
- Multiple air fluid level in case of intestinal obstruction.

Diagnostic Peritoneal Lavage (DPL)

When to use DPL?

- When FAST is not available.
- No trained personnel to perform FAST.
- The results of FAST are equivocal.

It helps in determining the presence of blood or enteric fluid due to intra-abdominal injury. The results are highly suggestive, but negative result does not rule out intra-abdominal injury.

When not to use DPL?

- When it is difficult to interpret in a hemodynamically unstable patient which cannot be sent to CT room.
- In pregnancy and previous abdominal surgery.

CT scan

- If needed, further to rule out other injuries, **with or without contrast when patient is stable.**
- Used to detect 76% of hollow viscus injuries, free air and intraperitoneal fluid, **retroperitoneal injuries** and helps in the decision for conservative treatment.
- Helical CT scan done to reduce the time in CT scan room, helical with contrast can detect arterial extravasation in blunt abdominal trauma.
- **CT reconstruction images are useful for detecting ruptured diaphragm.**

> Patient with *negative scan* must be observed often. *Repeat scan* if necessary.

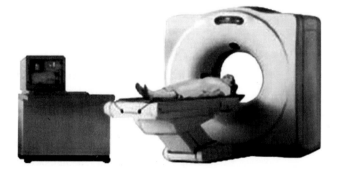

Fig. 6.19: CT scan

Focussed Assessment of Ultrasonography for Trauma (FAST)

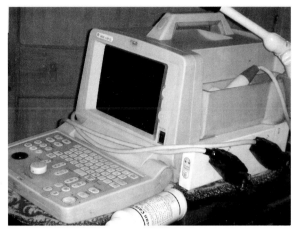

Fig. 6.20: Ultrasound

It is an eye to abdomen.

What are advantage?
- Quick, portable, easily available, bed side and accurate procedure done during resuscitation.
- Performed in hemodynamically unstable patient, who can't send to CT room.
- Great value and high sensitivity (100%) for detecting free fluid which accumulates in dependent areas around the liver, spleen, and pouch of Douglas.
- Very much useful in case of ileus, surgical emphysema under the skin to know free fluid.

What are Disadvantages?
- Unable to differentiate between blood, urine, bile, ascites.

Color Doppler
- Rule out aortic and vascular cause.
- Use to know measurement of blood flow.
- To differentiate cystic lesion from vascular structure.

How to treat?

Remember 4 'N' for any traumatic abdominal injuries.
- Nil by mouth
- Nasogastric tube

- Needle infusion—IV fluids
- Narcotics—IV analgesics

Tricks to be remember with mnemonics **"ADMIT"**
Activity (complete bed rest)
Diet (liquids or nil by mouth)
Medication (IV Antibiotics)
Investigation (repeat it at regularly interval)
TPR and vitals check frequently.

> Key for treatment is periodic evaluation.

- After ABC and stabilization of patient or in penetrating injury.
- Hollow organ (bladder, intestine) tend to rupture, releasing their contents into the surrounding space.
- Solid organ (liver, spleen) tend to tear, often bleed slowly enough that can be overlooked.

Surgical Management

- If free fluid with particularly organ damage.
- If possible, stabilize the patient with ABC's.
- Immediately go for exploratory laparotomy for control of bleeding with due risk and prognosis explain to patient relatives.
- Keep OT staff, blood transfusion, and team of experts ready.

Indication for Laparotomy

- Signs of peritonitis
- Ongoing shock and hemorrhage
- Deterioration of observed symptoms
- Free fluid findings in FAST.

Remember

Abdominal injuries are commonly seen in children and should be treated cautiously, as children can compensate significantly blood loss than adults without signs and symptoms of shock. Children can lose greater proportion of blood volume than adults can before symptoms of shock develops. What makes situation more dangerous is that children have less circulating blood volume thasn adults, so minimal loss can lead to shock.

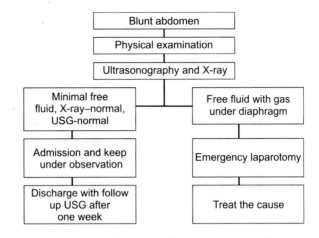

Fig. 6.21: Flow chart for management of abdominal injury

Prognosis

If not diagnosed promptly—worse out come.
Delayed treatment high mortality and morbidity.

Pelvic Injury

Pelvis in latin word for "basin", thus got its name from shape.
Fracture pelvis is usually life-threatening injuries.

Why Life-Threatening?

- High velocity injuries falling from a great height, crush injury or road traffic accident.
- Major vessels get torn off or rupture.
- Retroperitoneal hemorrhage.
- Patient can lose as much as 2 to 3 liters of blood in short span of time causing hemorrhagic shock.
- Bleeding in pelvis fracture is usually venous. Pelvic vein forms a massive thin walled venous plexus through which arteries intervened (Fig. 6.22).
- Injuries to pelvis can cause injuries to all structure in pelvic cavity like bladder, urethra, rectum, uterus.

   Sex—pelvic fracture more common in males than in females.

   95% pelvic fractures are minor, cited mortality rate for pelvic fracture are 3 to 20%.

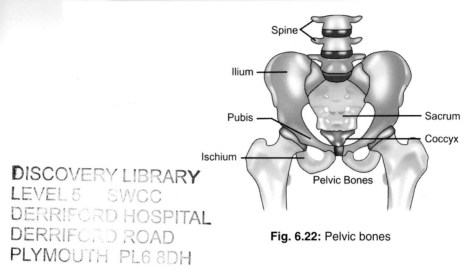

Fig. 6.22: Pelvic bones

Associated injuries, pulmonary emboli, infection are no exception adding injury to mortality.

Fracture of the outer pelvic rings not involving cavity, do not cause any threat of life.

Mechanism

Injuries usually sustain are:
• Compression from front to back.
• Compression from side to side—commonest injury.
• Vertical shear injuries—unstable.

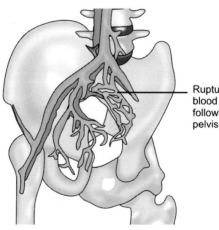

Fig. 6.23: Blood flow to plevis

How to Diagnose?

- History, mechanism of trauma.
- Pain in groin.
- Unable to weight bear, walk.
- Blood over urinary meatus present or hematuria—male more than female has urethral injury because of long urethra.
- Signs of shock.

On Examination

- Tenderness over pelvis.
- Pelvic compression and distraction test positive.

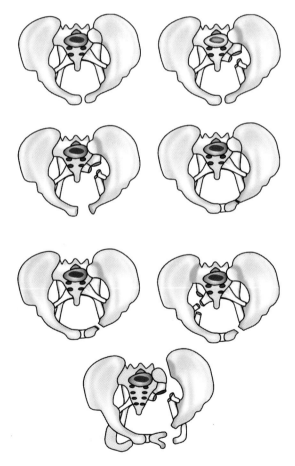

Fig. 6.24: Type of pelvic fracture

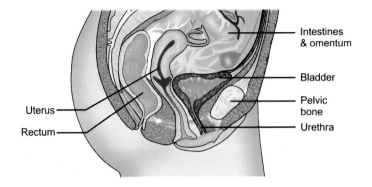

Uterus
Rectum
Intestines & omentum
Bladder
Pelvic bone
Urethra

Fig. 6.25: Cross-section of other viscera that can get injured

- To rule out hip fracture perform this simple test. Put fist between two knee and ask patient to squeeze the fist with knee. If pain elicits, pelvic fracture is present.
- Detail neurological examination.
- Routine perrectal and pervaginal examination.
- Rule out abdominal injury.

What to Investigate?

- X-ray—primarily used as key for early diagnosis.
- CT pelvis with 3D reconstruction are very helpful for acetabulum, vertical shear injuries.
- CT urethrogram or cystograms for urethral/bladder injury.
- USG of abdomen as mentioned above.
- Routine blood investigation.
- Angiogram for identifying arterial blood.

How to Manage?

Successful management of pelvic fracture depends on proper diagnosis and timely treatment.
- Acute
- Immediate
- Late

Decision maker or captain address the needs of damage control surgery (1993).

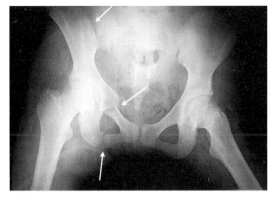

Fig. 6.26: Fracture pelvis

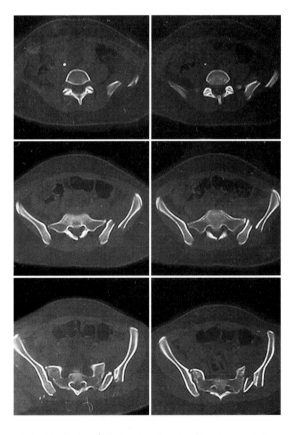

Fig. 6.27: Plain CT scan showing fracture pelvis

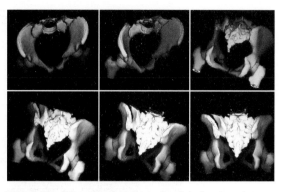

Fig. 6.28: 3D reconstruction of pelvic fracture images on CT scan

Take Care of First Things First

Tips and tricks

- *Pelvic traction*—to immobilize and decrease blood loss (Fig. 6.29).
- *Rapid IV infusion.*
- *Blood and blood products.*
- If associated injuries permits *early fixation of unstable pelvis with external fixator, to decrease blood loss.*
- Gentle manipulation should be done once as it will bleed more.
- *After external fixation,* (Fig. 6.30) if patient *stills remains hemodynamically unstable* then *embolization of bleeding site using an angiogram is done.*
- Rarely, *exploratory laparotomy* is performed to find source of bleeding.

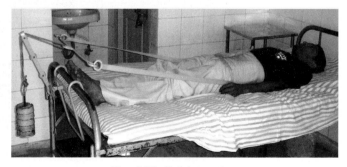

Fig. 6.29: Pelvic traction

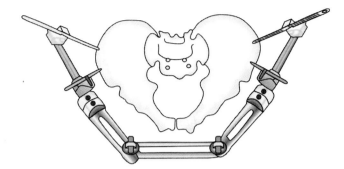

Fig. 6.30: External fixator for pelvis

- If embolization fails, **damage control surgery** like retroperitoneal packaging technique can be tried.
- Definitive surgery for pelvis can be taken care later on.

Do not place urethral catheter until urethral injury has been ruled out.

By physical examination or retrograde urethrography or until patient himself / herself passes clear urine.

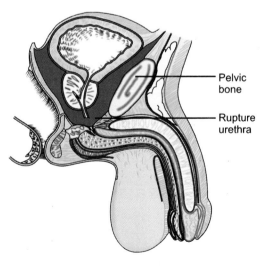

Pelvic bone

Rupture urethra

Fig. 6.31: Rupture urethra

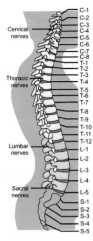

Spinal Injury

Back is a symbol of strength and hard work.

All head injuries and unconscious patient potentially have spinal injuries as well.

Injury to cervical spine C3-7 and the thoracolumbar junction T12- L1 are common.

Do you know you are dealing with unstable spine?

- History and mechanism of fall or accident (Fig. 6.32).
- Tingling, numbness over limbs unusual or absence of feeling or movement of limbs.
- Pain in back radiating to lower limbs.
- Unable to pass urine and stool.
- Tenderness over spine.

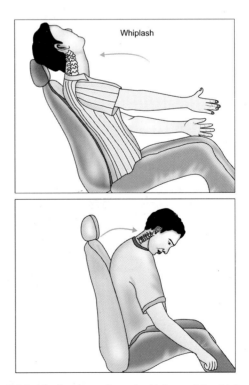

Fig. 6.32: Mechanism of cervical injury while driving car

On Examination

Utmost care should be taken to examine spine during trauma management, as you may further deteriorate the worsen condition.

Rapid Test to Know

> Can he move limbs equally strong? Can he feel pinch?

If any or all of mentioned tests/symptoms present indicates spine is unstable. Be cautious!

Inspection—look for movements, deformity in spine, wounds, urine/stool passed.

Palpation—look for tenderness over cervical, thoracolumbar junction, and lower lumbar spine. Look for deformity—gibbus, kyphus or any congenital condition.

Go for detail neurological examination to rule out level of injury, level of cord transaction.

Percussion—test to be performed by experts only.

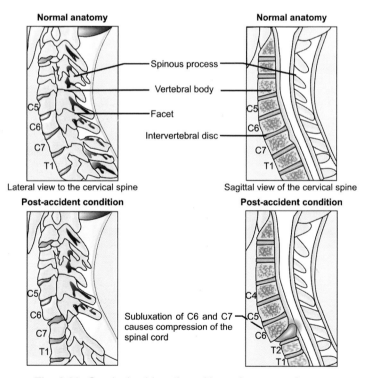

Fig. 6.33: Cervical subluxation with cord compression

Tip

> Don't test movement of spine.

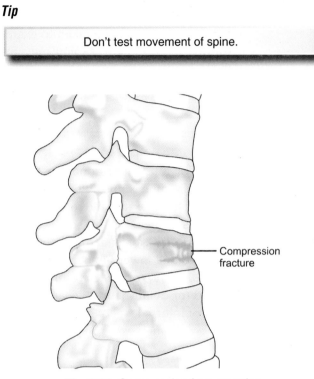

Fig. 6.34: Compression fracture spine

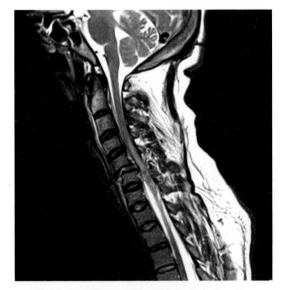

Fig. 6.35: MRI showing fracture dislocation with cord compression

Which are emergency diagnostic modalities to rule out spine injury?

As per ATLS, three screening radiographies are recommended during initial evaluation of trauma patient in emergency department.

An

- AP (anteroposterior) view of chest
- AP view of pelvis
- Lateral view of cervical spine.
- The goal is to screen out rapidly the need of emergency therapeutic intervention.

Management

- Head in neutral position—**not to pull or push.**
- Apply cervical collar and movements required using "logroll"method as mentioned earlier.
- Helmet removal priority, if not possible call expertise, if ABC is obstruction.
- Main objective to identify and stabilize the spinal injury to prevent ongoing insult to spinal cord.

Can you treat spinal cord injury? How?

Yes, on arrival in hospital and resuscitation is ongoing, medical management begins.

What is Aim?

Whatever procedsure you choose aim is to obtain free cord in stable spinal column.

Once it is stabilized whether to treat conservatively or surgically depends on experts—orthopedic surgeon. Objective is achieved by reduction, i.e. closed or open.

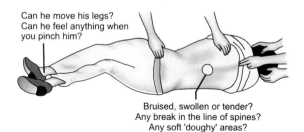

Can he move his legs?
Can he feel anything when you pinch him?

Bruised, swollen or tender?
Any break in the line of spines?
Any soft 'doughy' areas?

Fig. 6.36: Movement of legs and pinch, wound

What are the Goals of Conservative Management?

Is to prevent secondary cord injury which can be exacerated by hypotension, shock, hypoxia and hyperthermia.

Management protocols include:

- Maintenance of adequate blood pressure.
- Administration of steroid—mehtylpredni-solone given in a dose of 30 mg/kg intravenously over 45 minutes within 8 hours of injury in those with incomplete or suspected spinal cord injury. The initial dose is followed by 5.4 mg /kg/hr IV given over the next 23 hours by continuous drip. If patient begins treatment between 3 to 8 hours of post-injury, the steroid infusion may be extended to 48 hours to attain maximum benefit. However, it is still controversial.
- Aggressive pulmonary toilet, antibiotics.
- Catheterization—catheter, bladder care, regular interval urine examination and culture to prevent infection, urine output should be maintained 30 ml/hr.
- Stress duodenal and gastric ulcer should be prevented.
- Prevent hypothermia.
- Pass nasogastric tube if essential as ileus is common, aspiration pneumonitis in associated head injury in unconscious patient, antiemetic should be added.
- Immobilization in form of external orthosis in form of rigid cervical collar, halo fixation, SOMI ASHE brace, Minerva jacket, thoracolumbosacral orthotic (TLSO) (Figs 6.37 and 6.38).
- *Traction*—continuous cervical traction in flexion, extension or neutral position as per fracture dislocation. Skeletal traction in form of tongs if heavy traction is needed (Figs 6.39 and 6.40).
- Nursing care to prevent decubitus ulcer.
- Physical therapy to reduce complication like joint contracture and heterotopic ossification in paralyzed patient.
- To prevent risk of deep vein thrombosis and pulmonary embolism low molecular weight heparin should be instituted as soon as medically feasible.

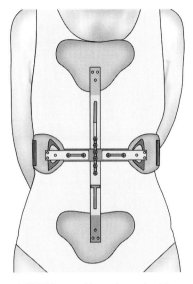

Fig. 6.37: ASHE brace (Anterior spinal hyperextension)

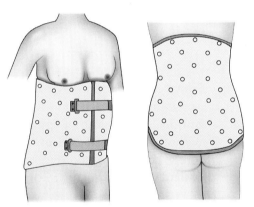

Fig. 6.38: Spinal jacket

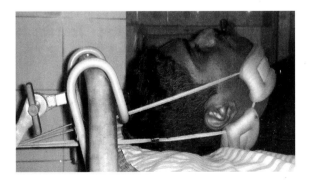

Fig. 6.39: Cervical traction

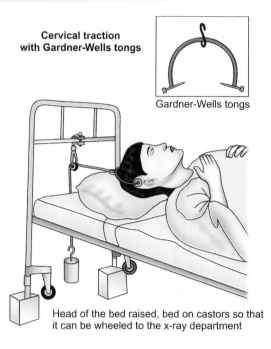

Cervical traction
with Gardner-Wells tongs

Gardner-Wells tongs

Head of the bed raised, bed on castors so that
it can be wheeled to the x-ray department

Fig. 6.40: Skull traction

Spinal canal clearance—drugs or decompression, drugs
as mentioned above and decompression by surgery.
Surgically—fixation of spine/fusion of spine with or
without bone graft and instrumentation like wiring,
screw, cage, plate, rod (Fig. 6.41). Never do surgery, if
patient is improving neurologically on skeletal traction.

Fracture

Bones have different functions in human body apart
from producing blood and blood cells through bone
marrow.

They have
- Protective function (skull)
- Supportive function (pelvis)
- For movements (finger)

So when bone is injured it will not only affect blood
production and function but can be associated with
muscle, tendon, nerves and blood vessels injury also.

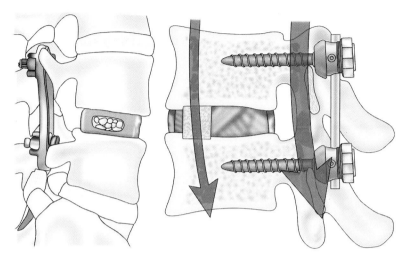

Fig. 6.41: Spinal fixation

Fractures can be

Open—fracture communicating with environment (it doesn't mean bone is protruding from skin) (Figs 6.42 and 6.43).

Closed—no external wound

Tips for How to Evaluate?

- History and mode of injury
- Pain over injured/fractured site
- Swelling

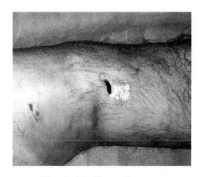

Fig. 6.42: Open fracture

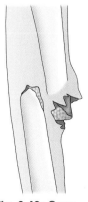

Fig. 6.43: Open fracture

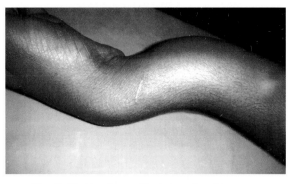

Fig. 6.44: Fracture with deformity of forearm

- Deformity
- Tenderness, Edema, Crepitus at fracture site
- Associated wound
- Distal neurovascular injury

How to investigate fractures—

For trauma patient its dictum "X-ray for everything that hurts".

Should not be taken during life-threatening situation.

Keep in mind for radiographic examination. "One view is of no view".

Tips on Examination

Inspection—look for open wound, soft tissue contusion, swelling, edema, deformity.

Palpation—details of wound, tenderness, edema, crepitus, movements of adjacent joint, distal neurovascular status.

Don't Crack the Treatment......Just Fix it

Stop active bleeding by direct pressure, rather than by tourniquet.

Tourniquet cannot be left by mistake, which can result in ischemic damage.

Tips and Tricks

- Initial treatment as mentioned in first aid
- Immediate reduction of fracture/dislocation, if compromise distal neurovascular status present with traction, splints.
- Preoperative planning of fracture by digital radiography has changed the scenario.

- Soft tissue injury should be considered seriously as it hampers circulation and resulting in infection and loss of limb.
- IV antibiotic and analgesia.
  Dislocation of any joint is an emergency
  It should be treated immediately.

Treatment of dislocation is usually by closed reduction with or without anesthesia. Rarely surgically open reduction is necessary. Post reduction it should be immobilized with traction or splints.

Fracture

Aim of fracture reduction is:

- *Anatomically* restoration of bone—to restore length, alignment and rotation, so that the joints above and below the fracture are in the correct position.
- *Stability* of Reduction—it should be gentle, atraumatic and sufficient stability should be achieved to get faster union and healing of bone.
- Early mobilization.
- To restore distal neurovascular status.

This can be achieved by either Conservatively in form of:

- Closed reduction and cast, spica
- Traction
- Pin and plaster.

Surgically by

- Open or closed reduction with
  - External fixation by rods, clamps, distractor
  - Internal fixation in form of plating, nailing.

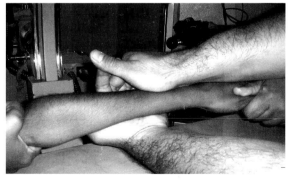

Fig. 6.45: Fracture reduction is done under anesthesia

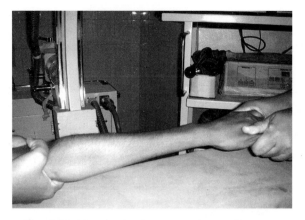

Fig. 6.46: Traction is given to get bony alignment

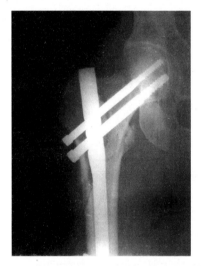

Fig. 6.47: Intramedullary nailing in subtrochanteric femur in elderly osteoporotic fracture

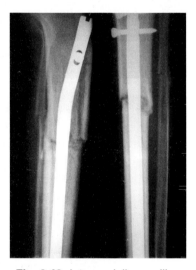

Fig. 6.48: Intramedullary nailing in tibia

Fractures in Elderly and Children

In elderly

Be aware of 'CHALKY BONES', in elderly osteoporosis.

- Elderly complaint of pain, inability to move limbs, suspect fracture first.
- To treat osteoporotic fracture is challenging for orthopedic surgeon.

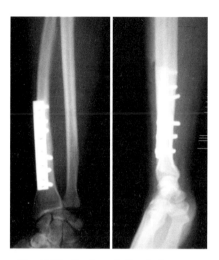

Fig. 6.49: Radius plating in forearm

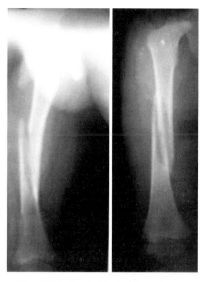

Fig. 6.50: Pediatric fracture femur

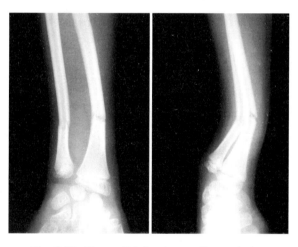

Fig. 6.51: Greenstick fracture radius and ulna

Young Children

- They are prone to fracture.
- Bones do not get harden for some years in children, so it tends to *'bend and splinter'*.
- Resulting into greenstick fracture.
- Treatment is to correct deformity and splinter by reduction and cast or surgery.

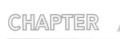

Specific Trauma Management

- ➲ Pediatric Trauma
- ➲ Geriatric Trauma
- ➲ Pregnancy Trauma
- ➲ Burns Trauma

Pediatric Trauma

- ❍ What is the Difference about Children?
- ❍ Primary Survey
- ❍ Airway and Breathing
  - • How to know Airway Obstruction?
  - • Management of Airway Obstruction
    - – Jaw Thrust
    - – Face Mask
    - – Bag and Mask Ventilation
    - – Oropharyngeal Airway
    - – Suction
    - – Intubation
- ❍ Circulation
  - • Why Children are Different?
  - • Management of Circulation
- ❍ Disability
- ❍ Environment and Exposure
  - • Why Children are Different?

○ Secondary Survey
  ◆ Head Injury
    ❖ How Head Injury Causes More Morbidity and Mortality in Children than in Adults?
    ❖ What Particular Assessment to be Done?
    ❖ How to Manage Head Injury?
  ◆ Chest Injury
    ❖ What is Different in Children?
    ❖ How to Manage Chest Injury?
  ◆ Abdominal Injury
    ❖ Why Children are Different?
    ❖ Management
  ◆ Spinal Injury
    ❖ Why Child Spine Kehaves Differently?
    ❖ Management of Spinal Injury
  ◆ Musculoskeletal Injury
    ❖ What's Different About Children?
    ❖ Management of Musculoskeletal Injury
○ Tertiary Survey

- Pediatric trauma is the commonest cause of death in childhood.
- Road traffic accident and fall account for 80% of pediatrics injuries.
- Penetrating injuries are less common in children.

What is the Difference about Children?

Children are having different anatomical, physiological and psychological characteristics than the adults which make children unique.

So pediatric trauma care also differs from that of adults, as children sustain different injury patterns.

Children are not Mini Adults

Anatomically
- Large head
- Small body size
- Elastic skeleton
- Airway characteristic
- Vital signs vary with age

Management

Treatment and management of children depends on age, weight and psychological needs of a child.

Remember

> Children are generally scared, so be calm and quiet.
> Be gentle (emotionally and physically).

Primary Survey

> Alert—encourage parents or caregiver to be present if possible.

As an adult ABCDE, early recognition and then correction for the underlying problem is important as children deteriorate rapidly. When assessing children be aware that they often *compensate* for there injuries by maintaining respiratory and circulatory effort. Ideally pediatric patients involved in major trauma should be placed on a cardiac monitor, receive supplemental oxygen and have constant reassessment of vital signs and oximetry.

Assessment

- Assessment should follow same principle as an adult.
- Weight can be estimated from age or head to toe length.

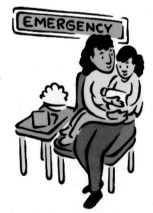

Fig. 7.1: Keep child with parents or caretaker

- Know weight of child to calculate fluid volumes and drug dosage.
- Management of patient depends on psychological needs.

> Don't forget to keep the child, warm -sweet pink.

Airway and Breathing

Assume that spinal cord injury without radiological assessment, exists in all trauma patients until proven otherwise.

Why are Children Different?

- Small oral cavity with large tongue.
- Large angle of jaw.
- Larynx is cephalad and anterior making vocal cord difficult to visualize.
- Trachea is short.
- Infants are obligatory nose breather upto six months of age.
- Diaphragmatic breather.

How to Know Airway Obstruction?

- Cyanosis
- Respiratory distress
- Use of accessory muscles
- Wheeze, stridor
- Dysphonia
- Low SpO_2

Management of Airway Obstruction

To immobilize cervical spine is the concurrent priority in all pediatric patients.

Clear airway obstruction as mentioned previously.

Be Aware

> Loose deciduous teeth, blood and vomitus may obstruct the airway so the clearance of the upper airway is a priority.
> Chest X-ray is indicated to exclude foreign body or dental fragments.

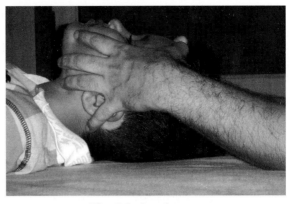

Fig. 7.2: Jaw thrust

Jaw Thrust

Indication—used to improve airway due to a child's shorter neck, small anterior larynx, short trachea, large tongue the jaw thrust maneuver.

Method—fingers behind the angles of the mandible bilaterally, lift the jaw towards the tip of nose (Fig. 7.2).

Technique is easier if the elbows of the person performing the jaw thrust resting on the bed or the surface the child is lying on.

Face Mask

Ideally face mask should be clear, so that you can see the child's skin color and possible presence of vomit.

Bag and Mask Ventilation

May need two operators.

Resuscitation bags used for ventilation of full term newly born infants, infants, and children should have a minimum volume of 450 to 500 ml.

Tips of Technique
- Fix appropriate size of mask to the bag.
- Apply the mask to the patients face, establishing a good seal (Fig. 7.3).
- Connect the oxygen tubing with 15 liters flow rate.
- Ensure equipment is functioning correctly.
- Assess effectiveness of ventilation then continue.

Oropharyngeal Airway

Indication—if jaw thrust fails to correct airway obstruction.

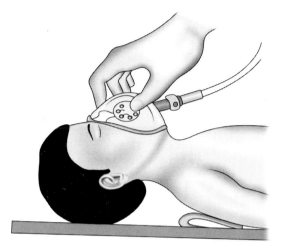

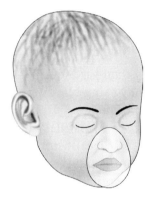

Fig. 7.3: Transparent face mask

Oxygenation needs to be optimized prior to intubation.

Sizing of oropharyngeal airway (Fig. 7.4).

Measure from the center of the incisors to the angle of the mandible, where laid on with face concave side up.

Procedure

Prelubricate with patient's own saliva or small amount of lubricating jelly.

Insertion—

• ≤ 8 years—insert under direct vision, concave side down, using a tongue depressor.

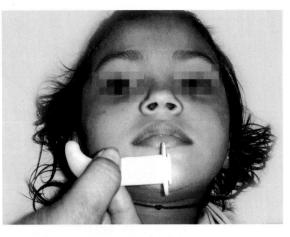

Fig. 7.4: Sizing of oropharyngeal airway

- ≥ 8 years—insert an adult size, concave side up, pass to back of palate then rotate 180 degree to concave side down.

Suction—if required, try not to touch mucosa, as this may cause bleeding and laryngospasm.

Intubation

When to intubate?

- Airway obstruction persist.
- Adequate ventilation not possible via bag and mask ventilation.
- Needs of definitive airway protection.
- Unresponsive to pain, GCS<8
- Neurologically flaccid, decerebrate/decorticate posturing.
- Needs prolong ventilation.
- Burns injury.

> In trauma oral intubation is always used.

> Under eight years of age—cuff tubes not used as it cause pressure necrosis on the narrow cricoid cartilage.

> Continue ventilating any child after cardiac arrest (including near drowning), even if they are breathing adequately.

Circulation

Why Children are Different?

• Normal vital signs vary with age

Pulse and BP according to age

Year	Pulse	Blood Pressure
0 – 1 Year	120 – 140 Per Minute	Systolic 70 – 90 mm Hg
2 – 5 Years	100 – 120 Per Minute	Systolic 80 – 90 mm Hg
5 – 12 Years	80 – 100 Per Minute	Systolic 90 –110 mm Hg

• Circulatory blood volume is dependent on child's size.
• Note - Actual blood volume is small— therefore small blood loss can cause   circulatory compromise.
• Children compensate large I/V losses (more than 30%) before becoming hypotensive.
• Hypotension is late and preterminal sign of shock in children.
• Metabolic needs of children is twice of adults because of:

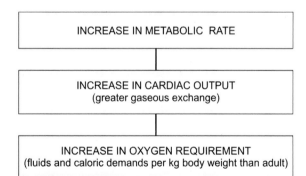

Fig. 7.5: Effects of metabolic needs in children

• Children are more susceptible to hypothermia due to their large body surface. Temperature must be monitored and maintained at all times.

Management of Circulation

Chest compression in infants
As mentioned in previous chapter, except following **tips** to be kept in mind.

Age	Landmark	Technique	Rate	Ratio of Compression
In infants	One finger breath below inter nipple line	Two finger depth – 1/3 of AP diameter of chest	100/min.	30:2 (one rescuer) 15:2 (two rescuer)
In 1 to 8 years of age	1 finger breath above xiphisternum	Heel of one hand, depth -1/3 AP diameter of chest	Same	Same
Older children 9 years till puberty.	2 finger breath above xiphisternum	Two hand over chest as in adult.	Same	Same

- Ensure adequate vascular access.

> Fluid boluses are pumped in so use large bore cannula or access.

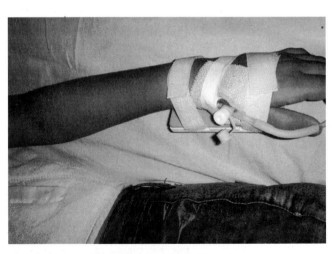

Fig. 7.6: Large bore cannula

> If intravenous access not available in 90 seconds go for intraosseous administration.

- Obtain blood specimen
- Assess and manage hemorrhage
  - Venous access in child is difficult.

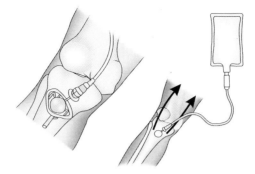

Fig. 7.7: Intraosseous administration

- Femoral or external jugular vein may be required.
- If percutaneous access fail.
  – Cephalic vein
  – Long saphenous vein
  – Intraosseous infusion may be used (Fig. 7.7).
- Control obvious hemorrhage by direct pressure.
- Splints and braces to stabilize fractures.

> Remember scalp may be major source of blood loss in children.

- Fluid resuscitation

> Fluid should be warm.
> Avoid unnecessary IV crystalloid fluid as head injury is more susceptible to cerebral edema in children.

- Hypoglycemia

> Check blood glucose frequently and give glucose.

Children have low stores of glucagons and high glucose required due to their high metabolic rate.

Hypoglycemia left untreated can lead to cardiovascular depression and permanent neurological injury.

- Drug administration
  If hypotension or signs of shock persist give packed cells or consider adrenaline.

- Reassessment
  Monitor
  - SpO$_2$
  - Respiratory rate
  - Heart rate
  - Capillary refill
  - Temperature
  - Blood pressure

> Circulation should be assessed by palpation of carotid, brachial or femoral pulse External cardiac compression should be commenced, if a pulse is not palpable or < 80 beats per minutes in an infant, 60 beats per minutes in young child or 40 beats per minutes in older child.

> Severe cardiorespiratory compromise in children is more often due to unrecognized hypoxia than unrecognized hemorrhage.

Disability

Neurologic deficit and screen

A — alert + GCS
V — Voice
P — Pain
U — Unresponsiveness

Glasgow coma scale is the best qualitative measure for conscious patient (as mentioned below).

Modified Glasgow coma scale is used for young infants.

Prognosis of trauma on basis of Glasgow coma scale.

Scale	Severity of head injury	Disability
3 – 5	Severe	Likelihood of permanent impairment
6 – 8	Moderate	Permanent impairment
≥ 8	Mild	Good outcome

Environment and Exposure

Completely expose with protection against hypothermia and hypoglycemia.

Why Children are Different?

- Infants upto 8 months of age have immature thermoregulation system, so unable to produce heat on shivering, it has to burn fat for thermogenesis, which increase oxygen consumption and vasoconstriction.
- Autonomic nervous system is not fully developed so ability to control body temperature according to environment is limited.
- Heat loss from head is more (18%) of total body surface.
- Less subcutaneous tissue for insulation.
- More body surface area, so children lose heat more through evaporation, conduction.
- To avoid hypothermia—use overhead heaters, blankets, warmed, humidified ventilation or patients body warmers.
- Temperature is usually measured axillary or rectally, but staff should be known that axillary temperature are one degree lower then rectal temperature.

Secondary Survey

It is more detailed systemic evaluation and initiation of diagnostic studies and is started after patient is stable and primary survey is completed. Use pneumonics.

History of A — allergies
M — medication
P — past history
L — last eat
E — events preceding injury

Head to toe examination—often common sites which are missed or overlooked during primary survey should be carefully looked for like scalp, neck, hands, back, perineum.

Head Injury

How head injury causes more morbidity and mortality in children than adults?

Because of

- Head body ratio is greater.
- Cranial bones thinner.
- Less myelinated
- Brain is less buoyant.

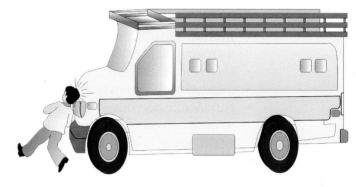

Fig. 7.8: Head injury following vehicular accident

Pediatric Glasgow Coma Scale

In children, who improve daily are most likely to recover while those who are vegetative for months are less likely to improve.

Age 4-15		Age < 4 years	
Eyes		*Eyes*	
Open spontaneously	4	Open spontaneously	4
Verbal command	3	React to speech	3
Pain	2	React to pain	2
No response	1	No response	1
Motor Response		*Motor Response*	
Obeys verbal command	6	Spontaneous or obeys verbal	
Localize pain	5	command	6
Withdraws from pain	4	Localizes pain	5
Abnormal flexion to pain	3	Withdraws from pain	4
Extends to pain	2	Decorticate posture to pain	3
No response	1	Decerebrate posture to pain	2
		No response	1
Verbal Response		*Verbal Response*	
Oriented	5	Smiles, interacts, follows	
Disoriented	4	objects	5
Inappropriate words	3	Crying interacts	
Incomprehensible sounds	2	Consolable inappropriate	4
No response	1	Sometimes consolable moaning	3
		Inconsolable irritable	2
		No response	1

What Particular Assessment to be done?

After primary survey, i.e. ABCDE is over and patient is better, go for it.

Secondary survey is done for detail examination.
- Look for missed wound over scalp, neck, back.
- Look for CSF leak, bleeding from ear ,nose to rule out fracture base skull.
- Periorbital ecchymosis (reckon eyes).
- Hyperflexion, extension injury to cervical spine without bony injury is commonly seen.
- Increase intracranial pressure.

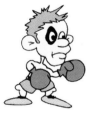

Clues to rise in Intracranial Pressure
- Decrease in Glasgow coma scales by two points or more.
- Changes in pupillary size and reaction to light.
- Respiratory abnormalities.

Tip

> Don't use nasogastric tube in head injury, it can cause intracranial infection.

How to Manage Head Injury in Children?

After investigating with X-ray—to rule out fracture, other bony abnormalities. If CT scan is available, it is the choice of investigation to know bony defects, hematoma, cerebral edema, midline shift.

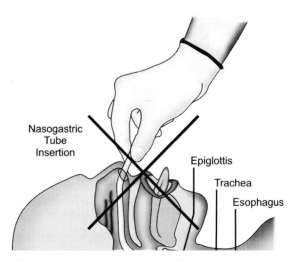

Nasogastric Tube Insertion

Epiglottis

Trachea

Esophagus

Fig. 7.9: Not to insert nasogastric tube in head injury

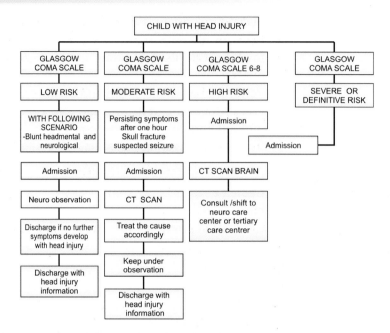

Fig. 7.10: Flow chart for head injury in children

Once diagnosis has reached,

- To keep it under observation in pediatric intensive care unit (PICU).
- Call subspeciaility.
- Supportive treatment and IV antibiotics.
- Seizure control with midazolam, phenytoin.
- Primary treatment is to control the elevated intracranial pressure by sedation, mannitol, fluid therapy, paralytics, steroids and CSF diversion (shunt). Induced hypothermia is a last resort to control elevated ICP.
- Second alternative is surgery—decompressive craniotomy.

Chest Injury

Rare pediatric injury

What is Difference in Children?

- As chest wall has elasticity and therefore major internal injuries may occur without any external chest wall injury.

- Mobility of mediastinum is less, so risk of major airway and vessel injury is decrease.
- Occult chest injury is common in children than in adult

    They are:
    - Pulmonary contusion, laceration
    - Intrapulmonary hemorrhage
    - Tracheobronchial tear
    - Myocardial contusion
    - Diaphragmatic rupture
    - Esophageal tear

How to Manage Chest Injury?

After primary survey with ABCDE and investigation, give

- High flow oxygen
- Analgesia
- Ventillatory support if necessary
- Insert chest drain
- Rest to part

Note: Hypoxia is most important feature of chest injury. Chest injury is rarely isolated usually being associated with other injury/system.

Abdominal Injury

- Blunt abdomen trauma following high speed acceleration-deceleration, direct blow to flank or back is commonly seen in children.
- Penetrating injury, gunshot are rare.

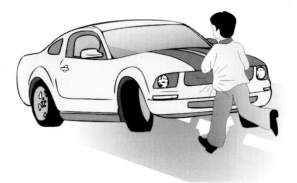

Fig. 7.11: Car or vehicle striking child's abdomen

Why Children are Different?

- In children the abdomen begins from the nipple.
- Less muscle and adipose tissue, so abdominal organs are closer to surface of body so less protection from ribs to liver and so more vulnerable to trauma.
- As children upto six years age breathe primarily with their diaphragms, peritoneal irritation from blood or intestinal contents may result in an alteration in breathing patterns.
- Due to small body size, injuring forces dissipate over a small body mass, resulting in a high frequency of multiple organ dysfunction syndrome (MODS) without ongoing signs of trauma.

Management

After primary survey ABCDE and investigate using FAST, give:

- Fluid resuscitation with 20 ml/kg normal saline.
- Second bolus, if required.
- If further bolus required, use blood.
- Immediate surgical reference.
- Pass orogastric tube.
- If free fluid is minimal treat conservatively with rest and supportive treatment and observation.
- If patient deteriorates go for surgical intervention.

> The vast majority of solid organ injuries (liver, spleen, pancreas, kidney) are treated conservatively.

> Children with history of significant trauma or high impact trauma should be admitted for observation even in the absence of signs and symptoms.

Spinal Injury

No examination of head injury is completed without spinal examination.

Rule out for spinal cord injury without any radiological abnormality, with objective sign of myelopathy as a result of trauma but with no evidence of fracture or ligamentous instability on plain X-ray or tomography.

Why Child Spine Behaves Differently?

- Vertebral ligaments are not strong enough to support the spinal column.
- Unstable atlanto—occipital joint, lead to AO dislocation.
- Because of relatively large head, relatively instability of the cervical spine particularly at C2 level is common.

> Hypoxia and hypotension are the most immediate threats to life and spinal cord function of patients with spinal cord injury.

Management

Important investigation to be done in emergency room is to take X-ray cervical spine—lateral, to rule out cervical spine injury.

- Immobilization with semi-rigid cervical collar, sandbags.
- High dose of steroids within eight hours of injury.
- Urinary catheter
- Anti emetic
- Usually treated conservatively, if deteriorates further in neurology go for fixation.

In child < 8 years-most cervical spine injuries (about 80%) occur in the C1-3 region.

In child > 8 years –most cervical spine injuries occur in lower three cervical vertebrae.

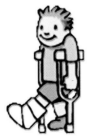

Musculoskeletal Injury

What's Different About Children?

- Bones are elastic, flexible, cartilaginous.
- Spine ligament quiet lax.
- Thick peristoneum and weak point is epiphyseal plate.
- Neck, paraspinal, paracervical muscles are weak.
- Elastic chest wall absorb high impact and transmit force to underlying structures, thereby damaging internal structure without external signs.
- Here everything is **smaller**, and sometimes small bone(ant) can bleed profusely (disturbs you).

Very Important is to Look for Fracture with Associated Injuries Like

- In children fracture of femur look for spleen or liver injury.
- In children fracture of humerus look for chest injury.
- Lumbar spine injury may be associated with pancreas or duodenal injury.

Management

After Primary survey ABCDE

- Immobilization/splinting
- Analgesic
- Clean and dress open wounds
- Antibiotics, tetanus prophylaxis
- Observation for neurovascular deficit
- X-ray of suspected part
- Nil by mouth
- Conservative—closed reduction and cast or spica.
- Surgery—fixation, in grossly displaced and unstable fracture.

Tertiary Survey

Should take place within 24 hours of injury, document any missed injuries, reexamine existing injury and their treatment.

IV injection for pain like narcotics are preferable then IM as variable absorption of the drug from the muscle in hypovalemia, cold or shocked situation and difficult to titrate once administer.

Geriatric Trauma

- What is Geriatric Age Group?
- Why is it Different?
- Goals of Trauma Management in Geriatrics
- Mechanism of Injury and Triage
- Assessment
- Potholes in Geriatric Management
- Treatment
- Specific Injury
  - Head Injury
  - Chest Injury

- Cardiac
- Gastrointestine
- Renal
- Musculoskeletal
- Immune System
○ Recent Advances and Summary

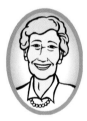

Over last 10 years geriatric trauma has become an increasingly important segment of injury.

As life expectancy has increased the trauma problems are becoming more and more in lime light.

There are several important principles to maximize survival and functional outcome in this special subset of patients.

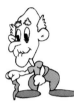

What is Geriatric Age Group?

It is difficult to stamp exact geriatric age group, but it can be summarized as once one's physiological reserves decreases and one of aging disease like cardiac, endocrine disease interferes the bodily function, one is geriatric.

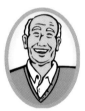

Why is it Different?

Because of increasing age, decrease physiologic reserve and higher incidence of preexisting medical conditions, utmost importance is given to geriatric trauma.

It is generally acknowledged that when the geriatric trauma patients sustain complication during their initial hospitalization it affects the outcome adversely.

So,

Prevention of complication is of utmost importance.

Physiologic reserves
Cardiac—Like coronary artery stenosis, systolic blood pressure generally increase with age, cardiac output declines with age, changes in cardiac output, decreased cardiac filling, diminished cardiac response to endogenous and exogenous catecholamine.

Renal—Kidney begins to lose nephron resulting in decreased glomerular filtration rate and creatinine clearance decrease.

Decrease thermoregulatory ability—hypo-thermia is increased risk.

Goals of Trauma Management in Geriatrics

> Not only to cure patient, but to make him live normal, independent, disability free life.

They are usually brought to emergency department by caretaker or family members.

Gather all possible information about the patient's past medical history, current illness, drugs taking, to make the best possible short term plan for caring of the patient.

- Be liberal in admission.
- Be liberal in radiological studies.
- Use invasive monitoring in high risk patient.

Mechanism of Injury and Triage

Trauma surgeon must incorporate the possible inciting event leading to trauma in elderly. More often the inciting events can be more significant to the patients course, e.g. syncope, hypoglycemia.

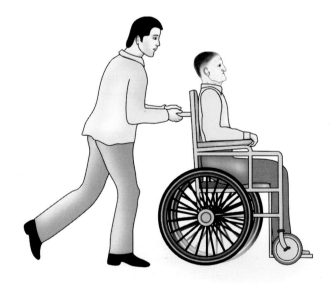

Fig. 7.12: Old people brought by relatives in wheel chair

Fall, pedestrian struck, elderly abuse is common cause of mechanism of injury.

Tip

To recognize occult injury that can kill the elderly patients.

Assessment

- Assess the scene and mechanism of injury.
- Monitor patient vital signs and over all condition thoroughly. Elderly patient will not be able to tolerate prolonged states of shock.
- Breathing and circulation priority as usual.
- Ventilator support may be needed.
- Complicating factors like facial fractures, dentures, decay tooth needs to remove.
- Face mask seal for rescue breaths.
- Expose the patient, avoid hypothermia.
- Do not overlook, deformity, abnormal noises (crepitus), bleeding.
- Assess neurological status.
- Transport and continue assessing neurological while transporting at every 5 to 10 min.

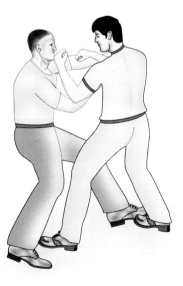

Fig. 7.13: Geriatric abuse by middle aged

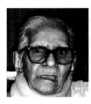

Several Potholes in Geriatric Management

- Neglected geriatrics—this is most neglected community by government, family and society
- Decrease in physiologic reserve with age make them less competent to fight against society, disease and trauma itself.
- One or more preexisting condition results in poor outcome of disease and trauma.
- Most of trauma centers currently do not have specialty centers for geriatric injury and different triage protocols for the elderly. The care of elderly in the prehospital phase should be modified as well.
- Under triage and over triage can be particularly lethal in geriatric patients. Avoid situation like "minor" results in under triage, which may lead to less aggressive treatment with poor outcomes.

Even simple isolated fracture can be life threatening in an elderly person. The loss of tissue tugor virtually affects elderly and produces significant blood loss into muscle compartment. Lack of cardiovascular reserve limits the heart ability to rapidly accept intravascular volume. Outcome at that point is likely to be poor particularly if patient has been under triage in emergency room.

Author's Recommendations

- Avoid exacerbation of any injuries. Elderly patient ability to compensate for injury through tachycardia and increase cardiac output may be impaired by medication (β blockers) and fluid replacement as soon as possible.
- Amount of fluid according to volume loss, patients condition—vitals, patients medical history—fluid should be monitored closely.
- Urinary catheterization .
- Intravenous fluids or infusion administered, vasopressor drug like dopamine or inotropic drug like dobutamine should be started, if the patient is in nonresponding stage shock.

- If systolic blood pressure remains low with dopamine, norepinephrine may be added.
- In acute myocardial depression with sepsis – dobutamine may be useful.
- Elderly with congestive cardiac failure may not be able to tolerate fluid boluses.
- If pulmonary embolism occurs—IV fluids and vasopressor used, heparin therapy if it is not contradicated is used. Massive pulmonary embolism is treated with thrombolytic therapy. If necessary, surgical embolectomy may be performed.
- Blood transfusion should be given if hypovolemia because of blood loss.
- Metabolic acidosis caused by lactic acidemia should be taken care off.

Specific Injury

Head Injury

Early **"aggressive care"** includes—endotracheal intubation for aiming protection, presenting with Glasgow coma scale ≤8, as traumatic brain injury in elderly patient more susceptible to hypoxia and hypotension.

Decrease brain mass, duramater adheres to skull and cerebral tissue shrinks resulting in increase subdural space and becomes more prone to injury.

Decreased blood flow results in decrease in cerebral perfusion and oxygenation.

- A bolus dose of 1 gm/kg of IV mannitol over 30 min may be given to severely injured head injury patient to reduce cerebral oedema, is still controversial.
- Diuretics may be added.
- If seizures present 15 mg/kg of phenytoin admininstered IV over 30 minutes and then by maintenance dose of phenytoin.
- All surface hematoma are to be evacuated with burr hole and craniotomy.

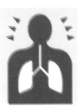

Chest Injury

> Geriatric trauma can likely lead to ARDS due to decreased chest wall compliance and reserve capacity as age increases.

COPD is common ailment in the elderly.

Chronic comorbid disease status, such as coronary artery disease, diabetes mellitus, renal disease can decrease physiologic reserve, results in hypoxia more quickly and less able to tolerate hypoxia than adult.

- Supplemented oxygen must be given.
- SpO_2 is monitor frequently.
- Rib fracture have low threshold for pain, so adoption of aggressive pain management strategy should be taken care with immobilization in form of belt and rest.

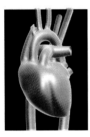

Cardiac

> Myocardium becomes thicker, resulting into reduced systolic function, resulting in decrease cardiac output and loss of left myocardium function.

- Fluid administration should be given with caution, as fluid overload may mimic preexisting disease condition like left ventricular failure, resulting into iatrogenic pulmonary edema.

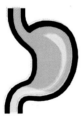

Gastrointestine

> Decrease in gastric motility, results in decrease water volume and results in imbalance in acid base metabolism.

- Water electrolyte imbalance occurs more frequently in geriatric, monitoring of electrolyte should be done and be treated accordingly.
- Exploratry laprotomy for penetrating injury, evisceration, peritoneal irritation are some of indication for same. Nowadays surgeons are more favorable with nonoperative treatment in blunt geriatric injuries.

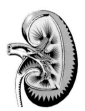

Renal

> Decrease in renal mass and vascularity changes resulting in compromising renal function.

- Electrolyte disturbance occur and decrease in urinary output.
- Diuretics, hyperkalemia, hypernatremia has to be treated accordingly.

Musculoskeletal Changes

> Decrease in height loss secondary to osteoporosis.

- Prevention of fall, and once osteoporotic fracture occurs its has to handle with care.
- Splints, braces and implants has to be chosen accordingly.

Immune System

> Impaired immune system, results in increase in infection and sepsis.

- Impact of infection can change outcome in geriatrics.
- As immune system decreases with age, judicious use of antibiotics is to be done to prevent further complication and septicemia, multiple organ dysfunction.
- Incidence of nasocomial infection is higher in elderly in turn results in a significant longer stay in hospital, subsequently increase in ICU stay, higher mortality.

> Avoid longer stay in hospital to prevent nasocomial infection.

What's New and What's Due in Geriatric Trauma

- The field of geriatric trauma is still in its infancy.
- Given the relation between advanced age, associated preexisting medical conditions and poor physiologic reserve, a poor outcome may be inevitable by the time the geriatric patient presents for medical help.

- Greater emphasis therefore should be given on injury prevention effort.
- Under triage remains a significant problem.

   While multiple clinical and demographic factors have demonstrated as association with outcome following trauma in geriatrics patient, the ability of any specific factor alone or in combination with other factor, to predict outcome is quite limited.
- Admission to ICU have been recommended, but its benefits remain unproven.

> An initial course of aggressive therapy seems warranted in all geriatric trauma patients.

Geriatric trauma patient, who do not respond to aggressive resuscitation efforts with a timely fashion are likely to have poor outcomes even with continued aggressive treatment.

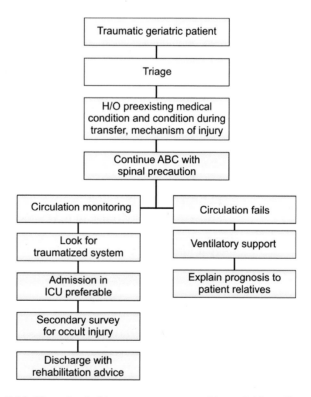

Fig. 7.14: Flow chart of trauma management in geriatric patient

Pregnancy Trauma

○ What is so Important of Assessment during Pregnancy?
○ Why Physiology?
  • Maternal Physiology Changes during Pregnancy
  • Fetal Physiology Changes during Pregnancy
○ Which are Diagnostic Modalities during Pregnancy?
○ How to Manage Traumatic Pregnant Patient?
  • Primary Survey
  • Secondary Survey
    ✧ Fetal Evaluation
    ✧ Maternal Evaluation
○ Pregnancy and Burns Injury

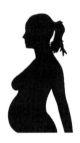

Trauma and similar violent events are the leading cause of death in young woman.

Although less than 10% of pregnant patient likely to face some type of physical trauma.

Trauma during pregnancy may be blunt or penetrating.

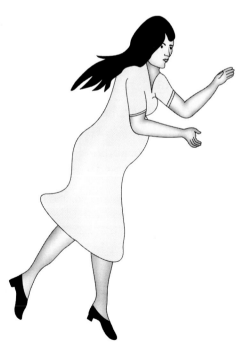

Fig. 7.15: Pregnant trauma following fall

What is so Important of Assessment during Pregnancy?

Resuscitation principles of injured pregnant patient are same as those for other traumatized patients with due consideration for specific anatomical and physiological changes during pregnancy. So a modified approach to the resuscitation process is taken into account.

> The main principle guiding therapy must be that resuscitating the mother will resuscitate the fetus.

What are the factors affecting trauma during pregnancy?
• Gestational age of fetus.
• Type and severity of trauma.
• Extent of disruption of normal uterus and fetal physiology.

Why Physiology?

Any woman of child bearing age with nausea and vomiting requires a history and physical examination performed in timely manner to rule out pregnancy.

An understanding of normal maternal and fetal physiology is important in the diagnosis, surgical management and postoperative care in pregnant trauma patient.

Maternal physiology changes during pregnancy

Increase in cardiac output and plasma volume up to 30 to 40% above the nonpregnant status in third trimester.

> Increase in plasma volume is more rapid than increase in red blood cell mass.

This relative hypervolemic state and hemodilution is protective for the mother because fewer red blood cells are lost during hemorrhage.

Despite of the increase in blood volume and cardiac output, patient is susceptible to hypotension for aortocaval compression in supine position.

Respiratory Changes

As uterus enlarges, the diaphragm rises about 4 cm and diameter of the chest enlarges by 2 cm, increasing substernal angle by 50%. Care should be taken for these anatomical changes when thoracic procedure like thoractomies are being performed.

The most important respiratory changes during pregnancy is in functional residual capacity (FRC). During second trimester **FRC is increase to 20%, counteracting 20% increase in oxygen consumption**.

30% of pregnant women have airway closure during normal tidal ventilation in supine position.

All these changes predispose to rapid fall in SpO_2 during apnea and airway obstruction. Hormonal and mechanical changes combine to produce hyperventilation.

Abdominal Changes

Increased level of progesterone and estrogen, inhibits gastrointestinal motility.

Decrease in competency of the gastroesophageal sphincter results in increase in chances of aspiration during resuscitation and surgery.

As uterus enlarges, it displaces the intestines upward and laterally stretching peritoneum and making the abdominal physical examination unreliable.

Renal Changes

As cardiovascular changes are reflected in renal system, increase in blood volume results in increase in renal plasma flow and increase in glomerular filtration rate, results in excretion of metabolic products (proteinuria, glycosuria).

Neurologic Changes

During pregnancy 25 to 40% decreases in anaesthetic requirement, i.e. even sedative doses result in loss of consciousness.

Coagulation Physiology

Pulmonary embolism is major cause of maternal death and injured woman is at maximum risk.

> Thrombosis is more likely to occur in pregnancy because of two components venous stasis and hypercoagulability.

Estrogen increases the hepatic production of coagulation factors.

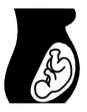

Fetal Physiology also Changes during Pregnancy

Do you know how?

The survival of fetus depends on adequate uterine perfusion and delivery of oxygen.

Uterine circulation has no autoregulation, which implies uterine blood flow is directly related to maternal system blood pressure. Once shock develops in mother, the chances of saving the fetus are about 20%. An abnormal fetal heart rate may be the first indication of a disruption of fetal hemostasis.

> An initial course of aggressive therapy seems warranted in all geriatric trauma patients.

Which are Diagnostic Modalities during Pregnancy?

Once the patient is stabilized and evaluation of maternal and fetal assessment completed thorough investigation to be done.

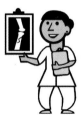

X-ray

Sensitivity to radiation is greater during intrauterine development.

> When performing radiographic evaluation of the mother, fetus radiation should be minimized by shielding the abdomen with lead apron.

In general X-ray beams aimed more than 10 cm away from fetus are not dangerous.

> Avoid exposure to radiation as much as possible.

Ultrasonography or 3D Doppler Study

- It is helpful but difficult to diagnose abdominal injury in traumatic injured pregnant patient. As fetal parts and enlarged uterus may interfere in evaluation.
- Uterus condition—rupture, tear, hematoma.
- Placental condition—location, abruption, hematoma.
- Fetal condition—viability and growth.

How to Manage Traumatic Pregnant Patient?

What are their Goals?

Goals

- Primary goal is to save both mother and fetus.
- Initial approach is same as pregnant and nonpregnant patients except minimum restrictions.
- Evaluation and stabilization of maternal injuries.
- Life-threatening maternal injuries should be given priority over attention to fetal assessment.

Primary Survey

As with other injured patient primary survey of injured pregnancy patient begins with same as ABC.

- Prioritize
- Resuscitation of mother according to ABCDE.
- Supplemental oxygen is essential to prevent maternal and fetal hypoxia.
- Severe trauma causes catecholamines to release, which causes uteroplacental vasoconstriction and compromise fetal circulation.

> Resuscitate in left lateral position to avoid aortocaval compression.

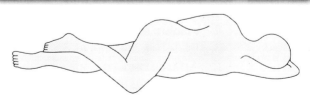

Fig. 7.16: Left lateral position in pregnancy

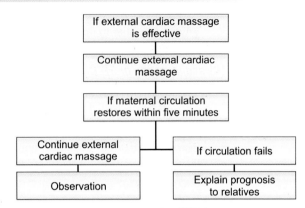

Fig. 7.17: Flow chart for CPR in pregnancy

Pregnant patient more than 20 weeks should not be left supine during initial assessment.

Left uterine displacement should be used by tilting backboard to left or manually displaced.

Continue doing CPR in left lateral position and do the following (Fig. 7.17).

Resuscitation of mother can save the baby. But there are times when the mother's life is at risk and the fetus may need to be sacrificed in order to save the mother.

Make a rapid evaluation of the general condition of the woman including vital signs (pulse, blood pressure, respiration, temperature).

If you suspect shock, immediately begin treatment, by rapid IV infusion with large bore cannula.

Hypovolemia should be suspected before it becomes apparent, as hypervolemia and hemodilution that may mask significant blood loss, so aggressive volume resuscitation is encouraged even for normotensive pregnant patient.

Secondary Survey

Aim

1. Determine gestational age.
2. Viablity of foetus as mentioned above.
3. To decide the plan of further management.

Apart from routine secondary survey obtain complete obstetric history performing physical examination in form of evaluating and monitoring the fetus.

Obstetric history is important to find out comorbid factors that may alter management decision, like history of preterm labor, any associated complication of the current or previous pregnancy.

On examination

Rapid method for estimating fetal age by determing uterine size, (Fig. 7.18) hence to know fetal maturity is an important factor in the decision and approach in pregnancy. Rough guide is when fundus of the uterus extends beyond the umbilicus, the fetus is potentially viable to external environment.

If pregnancy is less than 20 weeks, watch for abortion, bleeding P/V, pain abdomen, ectopic pregnancy .

If gestational age is more than 20 weeks, with bleeding per vaginum, consider placenta praevia **(don't do P/V)**, abruption placenta, uterine rupture.

Decision regarding continuation of pregnancy depends upon

- Stability of patient
- Approximate gestational age
- Availability of neonatal facilities.

Pervaginal and per-rectal examination is must to rule out for vaginal bleeding and cervical dilatation.

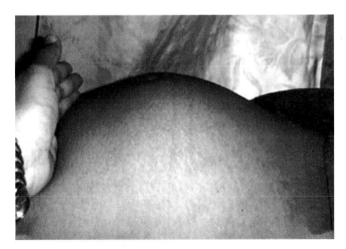

Fig. 7.18: Measuring uterine size

Fetal Evaluation

Begins with checking for fetal heart rate and movements at regular interval.

Normal fetal heart rate ranges from 120 to 140 beats/minute.

> Even if there is no obvious signs of abdominal injury because of direct impact it is necessary to follow frequent fetal heart rate monitoring.

High resolution ultrasonography and cardiotopographic monitoring seems to have the highest specificity. They should be instituted as soon as maternal resuscitative efforts completed.

Maternal Evaluation

Once the patient is stable, secondary survey begins:
Inspection of abdomen – for wound, bruise over abdomen, approx size of uterus. Pervaginal bleeding.
Palpation—determine size of uterus-gestational age.
Previous scar, scar tenderness, or any other tenderness.
Movements of fetus—more than 20 weeks.
Auscultation—fetal heart rate

The most common obstetrics sequelae after any trauma is uterine contractions.

Myometrium and decidual cells damaged by contusion or placental separation, release prostaglandin that stimulate uterine contraction. Majority of contraction (90%) stop spontaneously with rest and those contractions which are not self-limited are pathological in origin.

Placental abruption occurs in 2 to 4% minor and 50% major injuries.

It occurs as inelastic placental shears away from the elastic uterus during sudden deformation of the uterus. It occurs with little or no external signs of injury to abdominal wall.

Pervaginal bleeding, abdominal cramps, uterine tenderness, amniotic fluid leakage, maternal shock and change in fetal heart rate are indication for abruption placenta or placental separation.

Considering above changes occurring during pregnancy, manage and act accordingly to treat patient.

- Do first aid as mentioned.
- Procured ABC on site.
- Triage criteria is to be considered.
- On arrival in hospital, admission for observation even if minor or major trauma.
- If mother is stable hemodynamically, fetal well-being is to checked at regular interval.
- Discharge with follow up advice.
  - Fetal movements—in more than 20 weeks of pregnancy.
  - Bleeding pervaginal and pain in abdomen —in less than 20 weeks of pregnancy.
- In hemodynamically unstable mother, fetus is at highest risk of distress.

> Cesarean delivery should better be avoided when gestational age is less than 24 weeks, as fetus is too small to survive. However, more than 24 weeks emergency caesarean delivery will probably be favorable provided good neonatal set up.

Even slightest prolongation of foetal intrauterine life will probably improve the chances of fetal morbidity.

Pregnancy and Burns Injury

Treatment priority are the same when managing nonpregnant woman like maintenance of normal intravascular volume, avoidance of hypoxia, infection .

In cases of electrical burns fetal mortality is high (73%), even with low electric current. As fetus is floating in amniotic fluid, fetus develops "lack of resistance" to electrical shock.

Goals of management of burn pregnant woman are:

- Fluid replacement
- Respiratory support
- Initial wound care

Respiratory

Smoke inhalation is major cause of morbidity and mortality in burn patients. Carbon monoxide binds more effectively than oxygen. Carbon monoxide impairs the release of oxygen from oxyhemoglobin.

ABG (arterial blood gas) analysis, X-ray chest, and carboxymethemoglobin should be checked on initial treatment in burns patient.

Fluid

Fluid requirements are met with Ringer lactate. 50% of fluid is replaced in 1st eight hours and remaining during next 16 hours. Colloids (albumin) in 2nd 24 hours.

Fluid replacement is monitored clinically and by laboratory means.

Percentage of burns are calculated and treated accordingly.

Sepsis is another major risk to mother and fetus and is prevented by initial wound care, antibiotics.

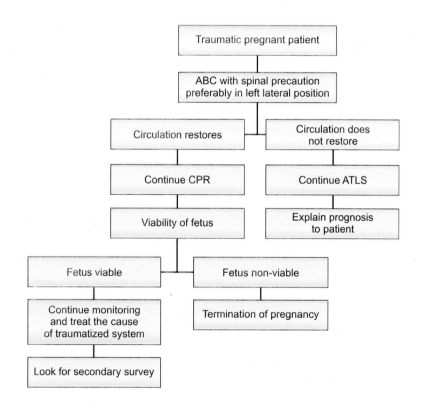

Fig. 7.19: Flow chart for pregnant trauma

Burns Trauma

- ○ How to Assess Burns Patient?
  - Primary Survey
  - Secondary Survey
    - How to Evaluate Burns Wound?
- ○ How to Manage Burns Wound?
  - Which Type of Burns should be Treated in Outpatient?
  - How and When to Treat Outpatient Burns Cases?
  - Which Burns Care Treated in Wards and When?
  - How to Treat in Wards Burns Patient?
- ○ What Happens if You don't Treat Burns Patient Properly?
- ○ Specific Burns
  - Inhalation Burns
  - Electrical Burns
  - Chemical Burns
- ○ Rehabilitation

Outcome of burns patients improved dramatically over last 20 years.

Because of awareness of people, education and advancement in technology, burns trauma is decreasing.

Mortality and morbidity following burns trauma is also reduced, because of early recog-nition and management of burns, availability of newer antibiotics, latest advancement in the field of surgery and wound healing method, scenario of burns has changed a lot.

Before management of the burn, wound care begins, the patient should be properly and completely assessed.

How to Assess Burns Patient?

Assessment of the burn patient is organized into a primary and secondary survey.

Primary Survey

Before starting assessment for burns patient,
Please, please don't forget to
- Remove patient from the exposed fire or electrical or chemical site.
- Cover with blanket or remove clothes in case of chemical burns.
- Immediately pour the cold tap water.

The emphasis of primary survey is more given on support of airway, gas exchange and circulatory stability. Early recognition of impending airway compromise, followed by prompt intubation can be life-saving. Obtain appropriate vascular access-central venous line particularly in large burns and place monitoring devices and then complete a systematic trauma survey including radiography and laboratory studies. Transport the patient to tertiary care center with ABC care.

Secondary Survey

How to Evaluate Burn Wound?

Once patient is hemodynamically stable and gas exchanges are ensured, evaluate burn wound in detail. Evaluate initially with extent, depth and circumferential component.

Decision regarding type of monitoring, wound care, hospitalization are based on this information.

Burns size and extent can be measured by many ways, but most commonly used is the "rule of nine". This is less accurate in children because of their body proportions are different from those of adults.

Burns depth are routinely underestimated during initial examination. Devitalized tissue may appear viable for some time after injury and some degree of progressive microvascular thrombosis is observed. Serial examination of burns wound is very useful.

Classification of burns depth

Degree of burns	1st degree	2nd degree	3rd degree	4th degree
Sign and symptoms	Red, dry, and painful	Red, wet and very painful	Leathery, dry, insensate and waxy	Deep involving subcutaneous tissue, tendon, bone
Characteristic	It can become 2nd degree burns with slough occurring next day.	Depth and affection towards formation of hypertropic scar is more.	Wound will not heal except by contraction and hypertropic scar.	Wound will not heal and mortality rate is very high.

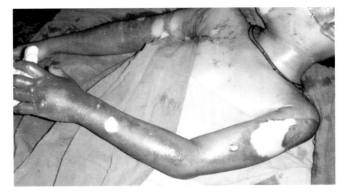

Fig. 7.20: Third degree burns with blisters

Circumferential component in burns

Apart from depth, note down circumferential and near circumferential burn wound because they may cause progressive ischemia.

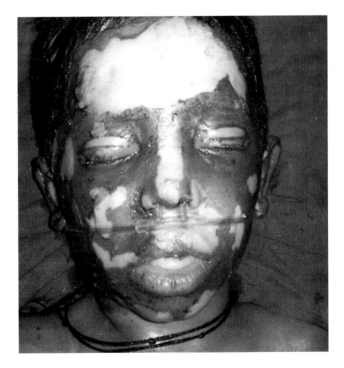

Fig. 7.21: Third degree facial burns

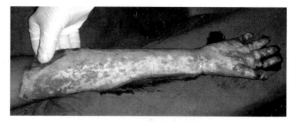

Fig. 7.22: Second degree burns

Timely escharotomy is essential.

Burns patient shows graded capillary leak, which increases with injury size, delay in initiation of resuscitation. Many formulas recommended by authors but most of formulas recommended that half of the total calculated 24 hours volume is administered in the first 8 hours post injury. After 8 hours, colloid administration is useful, generally albumin, 5% dextran. After 18 to 24 hours, capillary integrity generally returns and fluid administration should be decreased, following resuscitation endpoints.

> Generally burns over less than 15% of the body surface area are not associated with an extensive capillary leak.

Those who are able to take fluid by mouth may be given fluid by mouth.

> Electrolyte levels should be carefully monitored and corrected.

How to Manage Burns Patient?

Begins from site—as mentioned above remove patient from site, immediately shift patient to burn care center with ABC precaution.

On arrival in burns care center assess the burns wound after ABC is procured.

According to degree, depth, and extent of wound decide whether it is small or large burns wound.

Which Type of Burns should be Treated in Outpatient Basis and When?

Small wound can be treated on outpatient basis by expertise if it does not involve:
- Face, hand, genitalia, feet.
- Airway is not compromised.
- Fluid resuscitation not required.
- Patient is able to take adequate fluid intake.
- Patient and family must be able to support the outpatient care plan.
  Outpatient burns are usually 1st or 2nd degree and involves small nondanger areas.

How to Treat Outpatient Burns Cases?

On outpatient care plan
- *Wound cleaning*—with simple saline and removing debris and dirt, apply topical medication like silver sulfadiazine.
- Choice of topical dressing depends on surgeon to surgeon.
- Pain control by use of higher oral nonsteroidal analgesics like morphine, tramadol.
- Instruct patient and its relatives not to wet dressing, keep it clean.
- Provide cool environment by use of aircondition or aircooler.
- Elevation of the limb for edema.
- Beware of infection as in outpatient chances of infection are more, people neglect and don't care the wound. Give higher antibiotic.
- Always give all this advice in written with strict follow up dressing.
- Continue having long term follow up.

Which Burns are Treated in Ward and When?

- Large burns wound.
- 2nd, 3rd, or 4th degree burns.
- Involving sensitive area like face, external genitalia.
- Having more than 20% involvement of body surface area.
- Complication arising before and during treatment.

Large burns that require in-patient care by expertized once patient is stable hemodynamically.

How to Treat Indoor Burns Patient?

In-patient management

Management strategies for these patient are beyond the scope of this book.

Main principles of treatment are
- Initial evaluation and resuscitation.
- Initial wound excision and biologic closure.
- Definited wound closure.
- Rehabilitation and reconstruction.

Excision and grafting of full thickness wound otherwise prevent wound sepsis.

Skin substitutes, a number of membranes have been developed to effect permanent wound coverage, includes epidermal, dermal, composite substitution.

A wide range of *topical medication* is available from simple petroleum to various antibiotic containing ointments and aqueous solution and debridement enzyme.

> Always use silver sulfadiazine in initial wound care.

What Happen if you don't Treat Burn Wound Properly?

Burn wound infection-most common

According to **recent advances** in burns infection, it can be classified into:
- *Burns superficial infection*—loss of epithelium from previously epithelialized surface.
- Treatment—regular dressing of debris and exudate, topical antibiotic and grafting.
- *Burns related surgical wound infection* in surgically created wound that has not yet epithelialized with loss of graft.
- Treatment—regular dressing of debris and exudates, systemic and topical antibiotic and grafting.
- Burns wound cellulites—infection occurs surrounding injured wound.

    Treatment—systemic antibiotic and proper treatment of primary wound.

- *Invasive wound infection* occurs in unexcized burn and invades viable underlying tissue.

    Treatment—systemic antibiotics according to pathogen from tissue culture, wound excision with or without biological closure. This infection can be life-threatening. Aggressive combine treatment with surgery and antibiotics is recommended.
    - Functional or cosmetic damage.
    - Increase risk of cancer at the burn site.
    - Carbon monoxide poisoning.

Specific Burns

Inhalation Burns

- Diagnosis is primarily clinically and based on history of closed space exposure.
- Clinical consequences like upper airway edema, bronchospasm, small airway occlusion, infection, later on it can be ruled out by chest X-ray, bronchoscopy.
- The role of tracheostomy is controversial as it can be useful in prolonged intubation or thick secretion or difficult weaning.
- Avoid tracheostomy in children.

Electrical Burns

- Less common nowadays.
- Fractures, compartment syndrome, cardiac arrhythmia, or myoglobinuria is common.

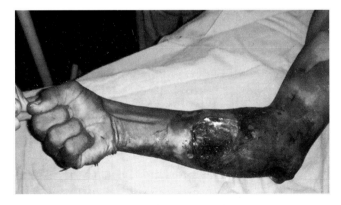

Fig. 7.23: Electrical burns

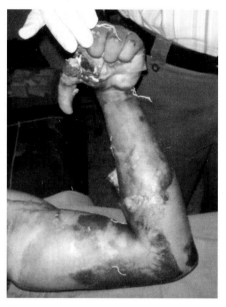

Fig. 7.24: Electrical burns with fracture

- Important first aid is
  - Switch off the power supply.
  - Remove patient from site with the help of nonconductive material like wooden stick, slippers.
  - ABC on site.
  - Transfer patient to burns or tertiary center
- Treat him once patient is stable as trauma pateint.

Chemical Burns

- Immediately removal of clothing and chemicals.
- Responders need to be protected themselves from injury. Copious irrigation with tap water should be performed for at least 30 minutes.
- Expertise personnel to be consulted.

Rehabilitation

This is final phase of burn care.

Tips

- Therapy should begin in critical care setting, including splinting, ranging, antideformity positioning. Passive range of movement of all joint prevents the occurrence of contractures.

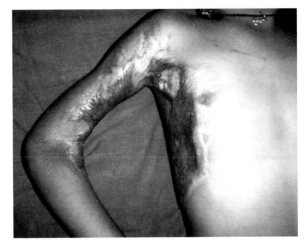

Fig. 7.25: Infected burns with contracture

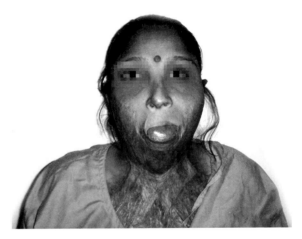

Fig. 7.26: Burns contracture

- Frequent change in position to prevent bed sores.
- Chest physiotherapy from critical care itself should be started.
- Pressure garment should be worn to prevent hypertropic scar, keloid.

With multidisciplinary burn after care program, most of patients have satisfactory long-term outcome.

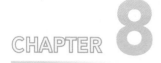

Rehabilitation in Trauma Management

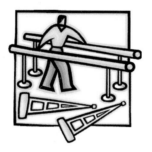

What is Rehabilitation?

Rehabilitation is a multidisciplinary continuum of services directed to persons with their disease and their families, usually by an interdisciplinary team of specialists with the goal of achieving and maintaining the individuals maximum level of independence and functioning in the community.

Does Rehabilitation Work?

Trauma Rehabilitation is a new field that there is little research specific to it.

It had been shown that patients where rehabilitation is offered, achieves a higher level of function than where rehabilitation is not available.

Why Rehabilitation in Trauma?

Trauma involves multidisciplinary treatment.

Sudden injuries causes patient to immobilized for weeks or months with potential complication for muscular, cardiovascular and other system, struggling with shock need not only physical rehabilitation but also psychosocial supports and time to work through emotional trauma.

It was developed to give people the support they need to recover their physical and emotional strength, and to rebuild their self esteem and confidence as they prepare to return to the community.

Once life threatening conditions have been ameliorated and the medical conditions stabilized, the trauma patient should be assessed for the restoration of maximal functional independence.

It is the role of the physiatrist and rehabilitation medicine team to identify, assess and promote the maximum restoration of physical, cognitive and psychological functioning of each patient.

Who are the Members of the Rehab Team?

- Dietician
- Physician

- Surgeon
- Nurse
- Occupational therapist
- Physical therapist
- Speech therapist
- Social workers
- School teachers

These all will provides their expertise in returning the patient to maximal independence function.

How Rehabilitation Works?

As a **first step**, it is important to identify the patient's functional deficit and subsequent level of disability and handicap as they relate to the patient's home, community, and school setting.

The rehabilitation process should begin early in the patient's critical care stay, because physical and occupational modalities may limit the adverse physiological effects of prolong immobilization.

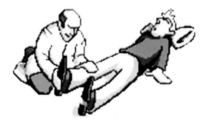

Rehabilitation begins from day zero with intervention includes
- Passive ROM
- Isometric strengthening
- Joint mobilization exercise
- Calf pumping,
- Appropriate bed positioning
- Suctioning
- Chest physiotherapy
- Orthotic devices placed at joints in a neutral position to limit contracture formation.
- Speech and occupational therapist can evaluate oral motor function assess safe swallowing and feeding to decrease the patient's risk of aspiration.

- The dietician evaluate the patient's nutritional status which providing recommendation for appropriate diet and caloric intake.
- The social worker and child life specialist provide the patient and family members with emotional and educational support during the patient's acute critical care stabilization.

Day two start advance system related physiotherapy like:

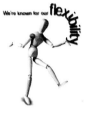

Tips in Neurological Condition

When patient is neurologically unstable, musculoskeletal intervention is not indicated.

Once neurologically stable, treatment is aimed at:

a. maintenance of passive range of joint movement
b. two joint/muscle stretches
c. maintaining anatomical alignment
d. inhibiting reflex activity by positioning
e. change of position will aid proprioceptive input.

Then rehabilitation is progressed to sitting and standing. This can be started while the patient is still requiring ventilatory support.

Tips in Head Injury

- During patient movement, the head must be maintain in midline position all times.
- During manual hyperinflation – small rapid breaths should be interspersed between hyperinflation to maintain the low pCO_2.
- Suction should be used when absolutely indicated as it has been well documented to dramatically increase intracranial pressure.
- It may be necessary to preoxygenate the unstable patient before suction.
- Before physiotherapy the patient's level of consciousness and sedation should be reviewed and an appropriate bolus of sedation may be given to prevent excessive rise in intracranial pressure.
- After a craniotomy if the bone flap is not replaced, the patient can be repositioned provided that pillows are arranged to prevent direct pressure on the unprotected drain.

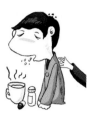

Tips in Chest Injury

- Support to chest wall to facilitate an effective coughing.
- Chest shaking or percussion are usually inappropriate, as patient will tend to " splint" their chest in response to any increase in discomfort and delay bone union may occur.
- Chest physical therapy – makes use of technique of coughing, suctioning, percussion, movement and drainage of lung secretion results in increase oxygenation

Tips in Abdominal Injury

- In adjunct to supportive rehabilitation, its rehabilitation starts after definitive treatment is over with
- Binders
- Abdominal muscle strengthening exercises
- Bladder exercises.

Tips in Pelvic Injury

As mentioned above, from the day one as patient is going to be bed ridden for longer period of time supportive therapy with importance and special emphasis on

- Frequent change in position to avoid bedsore in geriatric.
- Deep vein thrombosis and embolism should take care by calf pumping and chest physiotherapy.
- Joint mobilization for lower limb, muscle strengthening, bladder toning, positioning should take care of.

Tips in Spinal Injury

Patient is psychological breakdown stage with supportive therapy-give reassurance

- All joint mobilization exercise
- Chest therapy
- Back positioning
- Back muscle strengthening
- Bladder and perineal training
- Splints and braces to prevent deformity
- Gait training

Tips in Fracture

Initially start with soft tissue healing, i.e

- Muscle toning exercise with or without brace/splints.
- Calf pumping, chest therapy.
- Joint mobilization as early as possible to prevent contracture.
- Gait training.

What Rehabilitation Therapist should Know?

- How to organize and provide best possible care that is required.
- Familiar with injury and severity score predict outcome and risk of later disability .
- Risk factor for trauma related disability.

Future of Rehabilitation

It is still evolving and improving. There are many areas of research and improvement.

Evidence based treatment approaches understood and implemented.

HUMOR

Want to save a life?
Just do it! – Nike

Before going to save a life?
Believe in the best – BPL

If you are hesitating to saving life?
Vicks ki goli lo kich kich dur karo –Vicks

If you have doubt to save life?
Chances are 50-50 – Britannia

If patient slowly deteriorates!
Jor ka jhatka dhire se lage – Mirinda

Treat it with given tips and tricks
Likho script apna apna – Rotomac

If you succeed to save life
We dream because we do – Daewoo

After treatment, still not satisfy
Yeh dil mange more – Pepsi

If you satisfy?
The complete man – Raymonds

If you lost
Yeh sham ka sathi main our mera – Bagpiper

Index